Beyond the Blues

*Understanding and Treating
Prenatal and Postpartum
Depression & Anxiety*

Shoshana S. Bennett, PhD
Pec Indman, EdD, MFT

Untreed
Reads

Beyond the Blues: Understanding and Treating Prenatal and Postpartum Depression & Anxiety

By Shoshana S. Bennett, PhD and Pec Indman, EdD, MFT

Copyright 2015 by Shoshana S. Bennett, PhD and Pec Indman, EdD, MFT

Cover Copyright 2015 by Untreed Reads Publishing

Cover Design by Ginny Glass

ISBN-13: 978-1-61187-815-8

Also available in ebook format.

Previously published in print, 2003, 2006, 2010.

Published by Untreed Reads, LLC

506 Kansas Street, San Francisco, CA 94107

www.untreedreads.com

Printed in the United States of America.

Publisher's Note

The publisher does not have any control over and does not assume any responsibility for author or third-party websites or their content.

Praise for *Beyond the Blues*

"Shoshana and Pec have designed an easy-to-use format for all practitioners who work with childbearing women. While the topic is extremely complex, their book provides the most essential information in a concise manner. This is a long overdue contribution to the field of maternal mental health. Thank you Shoshana and Pec!"

—Jane Honikman, MS, Founder,
Postpartum Support International

"In *Beyond the Blues*, Bennett and Indman offer a compact yet surprisingly comprehensive manual on prenatal and postpartum depression. Readable and practical, they systematically address screening and assessment, finding a therapist, myths about nursing and bonding, and treatment. Interesting and helpful are suggestions for family and friends. For health professionals, there is detailed diagnostic and treatment information. *Beyond the Blues* is a quick read with an easy-to-handle format. Recommended for consumer health and health sciences collections."

—*Library Journal*

"As a nonprofit advocate and leader, my go-to book about maternal mental health disorders is *Beyond the Blues*. We promote the book through our work with hospitals, insurers, clinicians and advocates. Our followers find the book is a page-turner and provides just the right amount of information about maternal mental health disorders."

—Joy Burkhard, MBA, Founder and Director, 2020 Mom

"I love this book! It is easy to read and use as an informative reference for all aspects of perinatal mood and anxiety disorders. I recommend this book to all the OB care provider offices in my hospital system. It's an excellent book for my clients and required reading for providers I train. Thanks to Pec and Shoshana for the recent updates which make this great book even better."

—Birdie Gunyon Meyer, RN, MA
Coordinator, Perinatal Mood Disorders,
Indiana University Health

"Refreshingly easy to read and understand. Informative, concise and truly user friendly. A valuable tool for clinicians and consumers alike."

—Joyce A. Venis, RNC, Past President,
Depression After Delivery, Inc.,
Director of Nursing, Princeton Family Care Associates

"Succinct yet informative, a useful guide for the busy practitioner or overwhelmed mother."

—Valerie Raskin, MD, Psychiatrist,
Author of *This Isn't What I Expected* and
When Words Are Not Enough

"I lost my wife, Kristin Brooks Rossell, to suicide following a four-month battle with postpartum psychosis. All the things one should not do in the treatment of this deadly disease were done to Kristin. *Beyond the Blues* is a step-by-step guide that would have saved her life. *Beyond the Blues* is not long, yet its content is comprehensive and well written. I cried reading each page, knowing at each turn how this information could have been used to save Kristin, myself, and our families the pain and needless suffering we experienced."

—H. Reese Butler II

"An indispensable guide to understanding and treating prenatal and postpartum depression. This book is a gift not only to healthcare providers but also to family and friends of mothers suffering from these devastating perinatal mood disorders."

—**Cheryl Tatano Beck, DNSc, CNM, FAAN**
Professor, University of Connecticut, School of Nursing,
Coauthor of *Postpartum Depression Screening Scale*

"After reading *Beyond the Blues,* I immediately ordered several copies and shared them with colleagues. It is a wonderful resource, easy to read and full of practical wisdom. I've worked with postpartum families for many years and learned a great deal reading this book."

—**Maggie Muir, LMFT, IBCLC, Nursing Mothers Counsel**

"As a psychotherapist treating postpartum women, I have referred to the information in this book over and over. Drs. Indman and Bennett are two reliable sources who have checked all their facts while intelligently turning this very complex topic into something so clear and understandable."

—**Kim Richardson, MA, LCPC,**

"Provides practical, easy-to-follow advice for moms, dads, grandparents, and more. Most importantly, Shoshana and Pec paint a clear picture of this horrible illness. They provided me with a constant reminder that my wife was not alone in her suffering and would absolutely recover with proper care. The book provided hope at a time when it was hard to find."

—**Mark S.**

"*Beyond the Blues* by Shoshana Bennett and Pec Indman is a very insightful, concise, informative manual that should be in the hands of all providers and new mothers dealing with postpartum depression. It is a fantastic book containing all the necessary questions and answers."

—Shirley Halvorson, Past President,
Depression After Delivery (North Carolina)
Past Coordinator, Postpartum Support International
(North Carolina)

"This valuable treatment manual should be in the pocket of every practitioner who works with women. It is well researched and indexed for quick and easy reference by healthcare providers as well as clients and their families. As a registered nurse and lactation consultant, I have found it invaluable in assisting new mothers to comfortably achieve the breastfeeding experience they want with their babies. Thanks for dispelling so many of the old myths!"

—Pat Ross, RN, IBCLC, Kaiser Permanente

"Before I read this book I thought I was the only mother who felt this way. It was reassuring to know that I wasn't alone! My husband read the chapter for partners and he finally knew what to say to help me."

—Patty B.

"This book is an invaluable guide not only for women experiencing these disorders, but should also be mandatory reading for all who work with women during pregnancy and postpartum. It is a true breakthrough on the topic of prenatal and postpartum depression. This is the one book you should have on your shelf."

—Lisa Nakamura, Postpartum Doula,
Nurturing Mother Postpartum Services

"I never knew you could be depressed when you're pregnant. I was told that the pregnancy hormones would keep the depression away. I was severely depressed two months ago and my mother found *Beyond the Blues* for me. Now I am eight months pregnant, and I can't wait for my baby!"

—Carole B.

"I didn't know what to do when my wife started crying all the time after we came home from the hospital. The obstetrician handed me this book and finally things started making sense. It wasn't easy, but we made it through. The chapter for husbands was really useful for me because it told me what I should and shouldn't do to help my wife."

—Jeff B.

"Beyond the Blues is an informative and educational tool for ALL interested in gaining or enhancing their knowledge of prenatal and postpartum depression. Its simplified and direct approach is truly appreciated. As a mom and clinical social worker, I highly recommend this book. As a matter of fact, I already do!"

—Joy Fullhardt, LCSW, ACSW

This Book Is Dedicated To

Our children Elana, Aaron, Megan, and Emily for teaching us about being moms. And to our dear clients, who trust us with their deepest fears and greatest hopes.

Acknowledgments

With much appreciation to K.D Sullivan and Jay Hartman from Untreed Reads, who immediately understood the value of what *Beyond the Blues* offers. Sharon Cole, thank you for your fine editing eyes, and Ginny Glass for our new cover design. Thank you to Walker Karraa for her thoughtful input on doulas.

Shoshana S. Bennett, PhD
DrShosh@DrShosh.com
510-305-5040

Pec Indman, EdD, MFT
pec@beyondtheblues.com
408-255-1730

Contents

Foreword

This fine publication fills the education void between sufferers of postpartum disorders (women, men, and families) and healthcare professionals. Concise information is provided for all! Those of us who do clinical work and research in perinatal psychiatry define therapies, evaluate effects of medication for breastfeeding babies, explore preventive treatment, and much more—all very important endeavors. But the community of parents must be connected to well-informed professionals in order for even the most exciting of data to be put to use.

A very warm thank you to these two dedicated women for their commitment and sensitivity, and to Shoshana and Henry for their willingness to share the pain of their postpartum experience. It is my sincere hope that the countless people who read this book will benefit from your pain, thereby lessening the intensity of its memory.

Katherine L. Wisner, MD, MS

Norman and Helen Asher Professor of Psychiatry and Behavioral Sciences and Obstetrics and Gynecology

Director, Asher Center for the Study and Treatment of Depressive Disorders

Feinberg School of Medicine, Department of Psychiatry and Behavioral Sciences, Northwestern University

Preface

Prenatal and postpartum mood and anxiety disorders are very common. In the United States alone, over 3.5 million women give birth each year. Since the rate of perinatal (pregnancy through the first postpartum year) depression is about 20 percent, at least 700,000 of these women will become ill. The rate of gestational diabetes is between 1 and 3 percent, and the rate of a Down syndrome baby occurring in a thirty-five-year-old mother is 3 percent. Curiously, screening is routine for these conditions, yet screening for perinatal depression—which occurs in 1 in 5 mothers—is not.

While working in our communities, we have been asked numerous times to provide simple guidelines for assessment and treatment of perinatal mood and anxiety disorders. Mothers and their partners have been asking the question, "Why is this happening to us and what can we do about it?" Many good books and journal articles have already been written on this topic. Our main goal is to summarize the most current research and information into a practical, easy-to-use format.

This book is not meant to be used as a replacement for individual counseling, group support, or medical assessment, nor do we intend it to be a comprehensive textbook. *Beyond the Blues* will provide critical information for providers and families. Our intention is to offer the most essential and up-to-date assessment, treatment, and resources possible.

Introduction

Welcoming a new baby into a woman's life is like opening one of life's big doors of possibilities. Anything can happen. As healthcare providers, we do our best to help parents prepare for the birth, yet often gloss over the reality that bringing home a newborn with his own temperament and round-the-clock feeding will undoubtedly lead to a major life adjustment.

A mother must recover from her birth experience while her body undergoes a tremendous hormonal upheaval that rivals any roller coaster ride. Sleep deprivation alone can leave her stumbling around the house in a fog. She is also getting to know her newborn while confronting the loss of her previous life and any sense of control over her time.

Can this be overwhelming and lead to perinatal mental health problems? The answer is yes, and yet it's not hopeless. Perinatal mood and anxiety disorders are conditions that will go away with excellent help. Women, partners, and families do recover and are able to enjoy their lives fully. *Beyond the Blues, Understanding and Treating Prenatal and Postpartum Depression & Anxiety* is a resource that has helped countless healthcare providers, women, and their families to recognize the signs of postpartum depression and help those who are struggling.

Beyond the Blues is up to date with the most current research. It's easy to understand and offers practical, concise explanations. With a straightforward approach that brings the topic into the light, a range of effective solutions is discussed. *Beyond the Blues* also helps eliminate the stigma and shame that's been associated with perinatal illness. The support and guidance for moms, partners, and families is based on over forty years of combined experience by the two authors.

Beyond the Blues is an excellent resource for professionals and for those suffering. This book has assisted me in helping new parents when they're struggling. This is clearly the best mental health guide I've ever used in my practice. I'm so convinced of its value, I keep copies in my office to give away to those in need.

—Barbara Dehn, RN, MS, NP ("Nurse Barb")

One
Our Stories

We arrived at this professional focus by very different paths, one through personal suffering, the other through social activism.

Shoshana's Story

My husband Henry and I happily awaited the birth of our first child. We enjoyed a wonderful marriage and had planned carefully for the addition of children to our home. We had both grown up in healthy, stable families with solid value systems. We were well-educated people with successful careers: my husband, a human resources professional, and I, a special education teacher. I had worked with children for years, beginning with my first babysitting job at age 10.

I felt quite confident taking care of children. The picture I had of my future always included children of my own. I prided myself on being a self-reliant person, able to manage well even under difficult circumstances. Henry came from a family of five children and had always planned on having a large family. We had many well-thought-out plans for the future, and we looked forward with eager anticipation to being parents.

I felt terrific during pregnancy, both physically and emotionally. After childbirth classes, Henry and I felt prepared for the big event. There was one quick mention of C-sections and no mention at all about possible mood difficulties during pregnancy or after delivery. These classes were all about breathing techniques and what to pack in your hospital bag. On the top of every sheet on the note pad our teacher gave us appeared the words, "No drugs please." And it was also assumed, of course, that every woman would choose to breastfeed.

I endured five and a half days of prodromal labor (real labor, but unproductive), during which I could not sleep due to the discomfort. This was followed by another day of hard labor (still

1

prodromal). My baby was transverse (sideways) and posterior ("sunny side up"), a position that caused severe back labor as well. I writhed as the sledgehammer-like pain hit to the front, then with no break, hit to the back. After I hadn't slept for almost a week, my insides were so sore and exhausted I thought I would literally die. At that moment a very strange thing happened. I suddenly became aware that I was hovering over myself, watching myself in pain. Although at the time I had no words to label that bizarre sensation, I now know it to be called an out-of body experience. Still not dilating, I was finally given a C-section.

My illusion of being in control was shattered. I had been a professional dancer, and my body had always done what I had wanted it to. The visual image I repeatedly had during this ghastly time was of a beautiful, perfect, clear glass ball violently exploding into millions of pieces. That was the self I felt I was losing. Hopelessness and helplessness replaced my previous feelings of control and independence. I was left with a post-traumatic stress disorder that haunted me for years.

I soon learned a skill that I would practice for a very long time — acting. I bought into the myths that I was supposed to feel instant joy and fulfillment in my role as a mother, as well as an immediate emotional attachment to my baby. As my daughter, Elana, was placed in my arms, I managed to say all my lines correctly. "Hi, honey, I'm so happy you're finally here," I said, wanting to feel it. Inside, I was numb.

Overwhelming feelings, fear, and doom intensified as my first OB appointment approached. While I drove to the doctor's office, my anxiety level rose to unimaginable heights. I pulled my car over to the shoulder of the freeway. Hunched over the steering wheel, I experienced my first panic attack. When I returned home and called to apologize for missing my appointment, I perceived only a tone of annoyance.

I had lost all the baby weight in the hospital, but just four months postpartum, I was forty pounds overweight. I had always enjoyed a wonderful working relationship with my OB, and felt that he respected me as an intelligent patient. Now, coming to his office as a hand-wringing, depressed mess, I felt embarrassed and vulnerable. As I sat in the waiting room surrounded by mothers-to-be and women cuddling their newborns, my feelings of guilt intensified. I became totally convinced that I should never have become a mother.

Though my OB was well-meaning, his technician-like manner was anything but reassuring. He focused primarily on my incision, not my huge weight gain or uncontrolled crying. With tremendous shame, I confessed some of my feelings to him, including, "If life's going to be like this, I don't want to be here anymore." I was shocked and hurt when he leaned back in his chair, laughed, and said, "This is normal. All moms feel these blues." He gave me his home number so I could call his wife, but he provided no referral. As my ten-minute appointment came to a close, I began to experience my first serious suicidal thoughts.

I did call his wife, who was convinced my problem was that the baby was manipulating me. I just needed to put her on a schedule. I also reluctantly joined a new moms' group; since everyone was suggesting it, I decided to try. That was one of the most destructive actions I took. As I entered the room full of mothers cradling their babies with delight, I felt more alienated than ever.

Discussing "problems" in this group meant pondering the best way to remove formula stains from fabrics, managing spit-up, and calming a fussy baby. When I mentioned that I was having a bad time, an uncomfortable silence fell. I learned later that my name had been removed from the group's babysitting co-op. Upon leaving the first and only group session I attended, I felt more inadequate and scared than ever. Now I knew I was the worst mother that ever walked the planet.

Another complication was breastfeeding. Although my daughter latched on easily, I was overcome with pain due to inflammation and bleeding. I had been one of the "good" students who had prepared her nipples before birth, just as the nurses had suggested—rubbing them with a washcloth to toughen them up. I asked a leader from a prominent lactation organization to help me.

While the representative proved to be very helpful with suggestions about relieving the pains of breastfeeding, her emotional support immediately ended when I divulged that I would be going back to work in six months and would have to discontinue breastfeeding. She abruptly left my home. At this point I made the decision to stop breastfeeding completely, feeling like a total failure.

Life at home was frightening and unbearable. I had full-blown postpartum obsessive-compulsive disorder. Terrifying thoughts of harming my baby plagued me. I could imagine every household item possibly hurting my innocent child. Accidentally tossing my baby over the second-floor railing, dropping her into the fireplace, or putting her in the microwave were common worries. I would not trust myself to be alone with her. Not even my husband knew about these horrible thoughts—I could barely admit them to myself.

If I could sleep at all, I awoke in a full panic attack, wondering if I could survive another day. The simple act of watching television could turn an already dreary day into a deeper depression. The commercials portraying mothers in wavy white dresses, with naked babies in arms, taking delight in changing diapers and smiling angelically at their bundles of joy, sent me further into the depths. These were subtle reminders of the differences between all other mothers and me.

When my husband left for work, I would beg, "Don't leave me, I can't do this by myself!" He would return from work to find me in the same emotional state as when he left. I still remember my husband peering in the front window each night with that worried look, trying to see how many of us were crying. If it was just one, it was me.

Henry was frustrated with me. His mother, who had been a postpartum nurse for twenty years and who had popped out five babies of her own without the least dose of the "blues," was feeding Henry unhelpful information like, "Shoshana is a mother now. She needs to stop complaining and just do it." My respite came each evening as I tossed Henry the baby, proceeded to the driveway, jumped into the car, and sat and cried for a half hour. There was no laughter, no humor, no friends, and no plans. There was only despair.

My mother had come to stay with us for the first three weeks. She was wonderfully supportive, but even with her therapist background, she did not recognize the signs of this serious illness. For the next year I continued on my downward spiral. I allowed no emotional or physical connection with my husband. I continued to be deprived of sleep due to insomnia and anxiety, ate without experiencing much taste, and just went through the motions with my daughter. I felt buried alive with no chance of clawing my way to the surface. I saw a psychologist who never once requested any historical data on depression or anxiety in my family. All she did was probe for issues in my past, and if she couldn't find a real one, she would make one up. First she blamed my grandmother, then my sister. Finally she tried to convince me that having a cesarean delivery caused my condition. I ended up feeling "crazier" than I did before I saw her. I swore I would never again open up to another professional. When Elana was two and a half years old, my anxiety and depression began to lift significantly. "Maybe I can be a mother," I heard myself saying. My hair began to curl again for the first time since the birth. I began to enjoy my food and started seeing in color again, rather than shades of gray.

As with my first pregnancy, my second was flawless and without complication. I was enjoying my daughter by then, and the thought of a second child was a delight. After two days of prodromal labor, I decided on a C-section. The newfound enjoyment and relief from depression came to a crashing halt immediately after the birth of our son, Aaron. Although I could physically take care of him, my former "I'm incompetent" feelings returned. I would easily lose my temper at Elana, who was only

5

three and a half years old. Having been a teacher and knowing child development, I could not find words for my shame and guilt at the way I was treating her. The brief amount of time she had her mom "all there" was suddenly ripped away from her.

In 1987, when Aaron was almost a year old, Henry excitedly called me to look at a television documentary he was watching on postpartum depression. I was awestruck as the program described the disorder, its symptoms, causes, and possible cures. At the program's conclusion, I cried for an hour, looked at my husband, and said, "That's me!" The tremendous sensation of relief that someone had, at long last, described the turbulent agony I had been living felt like a weight being lifted from my whole body. Equally important, I had finally heard that postpartum depression is diagnosable and treatable and that it can go away! If this condition is so common, I thought, where are all of us? And why are we and our families being allowed to suffer without help from professionals?

I started reading everything I could get my hands on, from all over the world, and realized that many countries were light-years ahead of the United States in recognizing and treating postpartum mental health problems. In my research, I came across Jane Honikman, in Santa Barbara, founder of Postpartum Support International.

Jane generously offered me valuable information so that I could begin running a self-help group in the San Francisco Bay Area.

Although I was still depressed myself, I was excited about what I had been learning and wanted to share my knowledge with other sufferers and survivors. In contrast to the new-mothers' group I had attended, my group would be a safe place for women to discuss their depression and anxiety openly, without fear of judgment. I posted two flyers, one at a local supermarket, the other at my pediatrician's office. The response was thunderous! Calls came in from all over Northern California and some from as far away as

Hawaii. Every week my living room was filled with six to fifteen women, desperate for support and guidance.

I became convinced that postpartum illness needed the same support, psychological attention, and medical tools as other mental illnesses. This began my mission to begin a new career devoted to the study and treatment of postpartum mood and anxiety disorders.

For over twenty years, the support groups, which began in my living room, have continued and flourished. As a speaker, author, and psychologist I am joyfully continuing to pursue my life's work.

Pec's Story

For as long as I can remember, I have been interested in political, emotional, and sociological issues as they relate to women. In the 1970s I trained as a family practice physician assistant and worked in community-based family health clinics for a number of years. My interests varied, and my work took me to such places as women's clinics, an industry-based employee health center, a physical and fitness evaluation center, and weight management programs.

I entered a master's program in health psychology and then decided to continue with a doctorate in counseling, receiving my marriage and family therapy (MFT) license along the way. Many of my clients were referred by physicians, and much of my work with clients, particularly women, centered on issues related to health and emotional well-being.

One day, while in a physician's waiting room before a meeting, I came across a brochure from Postpartum Support International that described postpartum depression. I scribbled down the address, thinking, "I need to learn more about this." After receiving more information about PPD, I had a very mixed emotional response. I experienced sadness, extreme anger, frustration, and outrage. In all my years of training, I had learned nothing about perinatal mood disorders. I thought back to some of the women I had probably misdiagnosed. Why aren't health practitioners taught about PPD? My anger propelled me into action.

My second daughter was born when I was forty, after a workup for infertility, a laparoscopy, and a miscarriage, and thanks to Clomid. My pregnancies went well, but both girls, each at 8.5 pounds, were delivered by C-section. The births were positive experiences. My older daughter was able to rock her new sister in a rocking chair in the recovery room as my husband, parents, and brother celebrated. I did have the "blues," yet they passed each time as my incision healed. All in all, my pregnancies, births, and postpartum experiences were positive. This only added to my outrage when I learned about perinatal mood and anxiety disorders. All women should have the right to an emotionally and physically healthy pregnancy and postpartum experience! And all healthcare providers should be screening and treating them the same way they do gestational diabetes or any other perinatal health concern.

My history of political activism served me well. I joined organizations and read books, attended conferences and trainings. Jane Honikman of Postpartum Support International told me about a woman in the East Bay, Shoshana Bennett, who was doing postpartum work. I called and asked if she would meet with me to make sure I was on the right track. Since that time, I have been a coordinator for Postpartum Support International, and am a past chair of PSI's Education and Training Committee. I have created curriculum, lectured and given trainings all over the United States, and been honored to give keynote talks in Beijing and Shanghai, China. I have served as a consultant for both federal and local governmental perinatal programs. As part of PSI's educational committee, I am delighted to have been involved in the creation of our first educational DVD, *Healthy Mom, Happy Family* (see the Resources section).

This work has become my passion. I have never experienced so much personal and professional meaning and reward. I hope you will join us on this mission.

Two
Perinatal Psychiatric Illness

Some of the words or terms we use are medically based. We have included an Appendix in the back of the book to clarify and explain the meanings of these words.

Perinatal mood and anxiety disorders (PMADs) occur during pregnancy and the first year after a woman gives birth. The terms *prenatal* (during pregnancy) and *postpartum* (after birth) are also used to describe more specifically when these conditions occur. These mood and anxiety disorders are triggered mainly by hormonal changes, which then affect brain chemicals called neurotransmitters. Life stressors, such as moving, illness, poor partner support, financial problems, and social isolation, are certainly also important and will negatively affect the woman's mental state. Strong emotional, social, and physical support will help her recovery.

Perinatal mood and anxiety disorders behave quite differently from other mood or anxiety disorders experienced at other times, because the hormones are going up and down. A woman with a PMAD often feels as if she's "losing it," since she can never predict how she will feel at any given moment. For instance, at 8:00 am, she may be gripped with anxiety, at 10:00 am feel almost normal, and at 10:30 am become depressed.

Our clients who have had personal histories of depression tell us that perinatal depression feels very different from (and usually much worse than) depressions at other times in their lives. One of Shoshana's postpartum clients is a survivor of breast cancer. At a support group, she beautifully explained:

When I had cancer, I thought that was the worst experience I could ever have. I was wrong—this is. With cancer, I allowed myself to ask for and receive help, and expected to be depressed. My friends and family rallied around me, bringing me meals, cleaning my house, and giving me

9

lots of emotional support. Now, during postpartum depression, I feel guilty asking for help and ashamed of my depression. Everyone expects me to feel happy and doesn't accept that this illness is just as real as cancer.

Women who experience these symptoms need to speak up and be persistent in getting proper care. In the past, these illnesses have been downplayed and even dismissed. Research has shown how important it is to treat perinatal mood and anxiety disorders for the health and well-being of the mother, baby, and entire family.

Perinatal Mood and Anxiety Disorders

There are six principal perinatal mood and anxiety disorders, which are

- Depression
- Obsessive-compulsive disorder (OCD)
- Panic disorder
- Psychosis
- Post-traumatic stress disorder (PTSD)
- Bipolar disorder I or II (sometimes referred to as Bipolar Spectrum Disorder)

This chapter explains each of these disorders, some of their most common symptoms, and risk factors. It is important to note that symptoms and their severity can change over the course of an illness. Also, when "personal or family history" is listed as a high risk factor, be aware that often relatives with these conditions may not have been formally diagnosed or treated.

The Psychiatric Issues of Pregnancy

Contrary to popular mythology, pregnancy is not always a happy, glowing experience. Pregnant women can and do experience depression, bipolar disorder, anxiety and panic, post-traumatic stress disorder, obsessive-compulsive disorder, and even psychosis. This may be a reoccurrence of a previous illness, or a new onset of illness. Approximately 15 to 23 percent of pregnant women experience depression. These rates are even higher in teenagers and poor women. Risk factors associated with prenatal depression include life stress, a history of depression, lack of social support, domestic violence, and unplanned pregnancy.

In a 2013 study of 10,000 new mothers, it was found that 26.5 percent had histories of depression before pregnancy, 33.4 percent had their first occurrence of depression during pregnancy, and 40.1 percent developed postpartum depression as their first depression.

It can be confusing that many of the normal symptoms of pregnancy are very similar to symptoms of depression. It is easy to ignore or dismiss these symptoms as just a normal part of pregnancy. It is important that symptoms be evaluated and treated, if they are outside the normal range. The following section provides some guidelines to determine if symptoms are caused by pregnancy or depression.

PREGNANCY	DEPRESSION
Mood up and down, teary	Mood mostly down, gloomy, hopeless
Self-esteem unchanged	Low self-esteem, guilt
Can fall asleep, physical problems may waken (bladder, heartburn), can fall back to sleep	May have trouble falling asleep, may have early morning wakening and difficulty falling back to sleep
Tires easily, rest refreshes and energizes	Rest does not help reduce fatigue
Feels pleasure, joy, and anticipation	Lack of joy or pleasure
Appetite increases	Appetite may decrease

Depression and Anxiety in Pregnancy

When symptoms of depression or other mood or anxiety disorders make it difficult to function on a day-to-day basis, treatment is necessary. This may include traditional (counseling and medication) or nontraditional methods (such as yoga or acupuncture), or any combination. What's important is to use whatever works best, so you feel like yourself again. Depression during pregnancy has been associated with low birth weight (less than 5.5 pounds) and preterm delivery (less than thirty-seven weeks). Severe anxiety during pregnancy may cause harm to a growing fetus. This is partly because cortisol, a hormone released during stress, can cause constriction of the blood vessels in the placenta.

Some women become pregnant while taking medications for depression, anxiety, and other mood problems. Many of these medications are considered acceptable during pregnancy, if necessary to keep the woman well. Seek out a healthcare practitioner who is familiar with the current research about the safety of taking medications during pregnancy. Do not assume all healthcare providers are informed or up to date about treating mood or anxiety problems during pregnancy (refer to "Finding a Therapist or Medical Practitioner" in Chapter 3).

The rate of relapse for a major depressive disorder (MDD) in women who discontinue their medication before conception is between 50 and 75 percent. In other words, only 25 to 50 percent of women who stopped taking medication before trying to get pregnant stayed well. The rate of relapse for MDD, in those who discontinue medications at conception or in early pregnancy, is 75 percent with up to 60 percent relapsing in the first trimester. This means that most of the women who stopped medication once they discovered they were pregnant became ill again. In one study, 42 percent of women who discontinued medications at conception resumed medications at some time during their pregnancy. Resources listed at the end of this book provide helpful guidelines regarding the use of medications. Important factors to know:

- Depression and anxiety occur in 15 to 23 percent of pregnant women
- Higher rates are seen in teens and women of color.
- Onset can occur any time during the pregnancy.

Symptoms of Depression and Anxiety

- Sad mood
- Irritability

- Lack of joy or pleasure, not looking forward to the future
- Guilt
- Excessive worry or fear
- Social withdrawal
- Appetite and sleep disturbances

Risk Factors

- Personal or family history of mental health problems (diagnosed or not)
- Lack of support
- Stopping psychiatric medication
- History of abuse, domestic violence
- History of pregnancy loss

Stacey's Story

I had always wanted to be a mom. I was the oldest of four and took care of my brothers and sisters. We were all verbally abused, and I was treated for depression in high school and in my twenties. When I got pregnant, I immediately stopped my medication. It was a terrible pregnancy, and I became very depressed. I didn't eat well, I didn't feel like shopping for baby things, I didn't feel any of the joy and excitement I thought I would feel. I felt like I wouldn't be able to be a good mom and that I'd made a big mistake.

Finally, after being diagnosed with postpartum depression, I went back on medication. I began to feel better, shop for the baby, and most importantly enjoy her. "When I wanted to get pregnant again, I consulted a psychiatrist trained in issues related to medications in pregnancy. Together we discussed the risks of being on medication compared to the risks to me, the baby, and my toddler if I went off medication and became depressed again. I decided to stay on the medication during the pregnancy. It was very different the second time. I really bonded with the baby growing inside me, and could enjoy him (and his sister) after he was born. I really wish I could've enjoyed the first pregnancy.

After the Birth, "Baby Blues" — Not a Disorder

The term *Baby Blues* is used to describe *mild* mood swings that occur the first few weeks after birth. This is not considered a disorder since the majority of mothers experience it. Baby Blues:

- Occurs in about 80 percent of mothers
- Begins during first week postpartum
- Should be gone by three weeks postpartum

Symptoms

- Moodiness
- Crying
- Sadness
- Worry
- Lack of concentration
- Forgetfulness
- Feelings of dependency

Causes

- Rapid hormonal changes
- Physical and emotional stress of birthing
- Physical discomforts
- Emotional letdown after pregnancy and birth
- Awareness and fear about increased responsibility
- Fatigue and sleep deprivation
- Disappointments including the birth, partner support, nursing, and the baby

Deborah's Story

For about a week and a half after my baby was born I would cry for no reason at all. Sometimes I would feel overwhelmed, especially when I was up at night with my son. Once I even thought that I had made a big mistake having a child. I felt resentment toward my husband since his life stayed pretty much the same and mine was turned upside down. When I started going to the mother's club at two weeks, I felt so relieved that all these other moms felt the same way.

Deborah's Treatment

Since Deborah was experiencing normal postpartum adjustment, she did not require any formal treatment. All she needed in order to enjoy her new life was a combination of socializing with other moms, more sleep, taking time to care for herself, and working out a plan of sharing child and household responsibilities with her husband.

Depression and Anxiety Postpartum

This section describes depression and anxiety that occur postpartum, which means after a woman gives birth.

- It occurs in 15 to 20 percent of mothers.
- Onset is usually gradual, but it can be rapid and begin any time in the first year.

Symptoms May Include

- Excessive worry or fear
- Irritability or short temper
- Feeling overwhelmed and unable to cope
- Difficulty making decisions
- Sadness
- Hopelessness
- Feelings of guilt
- Sleep problems (often the woman cannot sleep or sleeps too much), fatigue
- Physical symptoms or complaints without apparent physical cause
- Discomfort around the baby or a lack of feeling toward the baby
- Loss of focus and concentration (may miss appointments, for example)
- Loss of interest or pleasure, lower sex drive
- Changes in appetite, significant weight loss or gain

Risk Factors

- From 50 to 80 percent risk if previous postpartum depression/anxiety
- Depression or anxiety during pregnancy
- Personal or family history of depression/anxiety
- Abrupt weaning
- Social isolation or poor support
- History of premenstrual syndrome (PMS) or premenstrual dysphoric disorder (PMDD)
- Negative mood changes while taking birth control pills or fertility medication
- Thyroid dysfunction
- Stopping psychiatric medication

Lori's Story

I was so excited about having our baby girl. My pregnancy had gone smoothly. I had been warned about the "Blues," but I just couldn't shake the tears and sadness that seemed to get deeper and darker every day. My appetite was nonexistent, although I forced myself to eat because I was nursing. I lost about thirty pounds the first month. At night I was having trouble sleeping. My husband and baby would be asleep but I would have one worry after another going through my head. I was exhausted. I felt like my brain had been kidnapped. I couldn't make decisions, couldn't focus, and didn't want to be left alone with the baby.

I wanted to run away. I withdrew from friends and felt guilty about not returning phone calls, emails or texts. I couldn't understand why I felt so bad; I had the greatest, most supportive husband, a home I loved, and the beautiful baby I had always wanted. At times I felt close to her, but at other times I felt like I was just going through the motions—she could have been someone else's child. I thought I was the worst mother and wife on the face of the earth.

Lori's Treatment

Lori began psychotherapy and also saw a psychiatrist for medication. She was started on an antidepressant, and the dosage was gradually increased. Initially she took medication to help her sleep as well. She began taking regular breaks to take care of herself. She also started attending a postpartum depression support group and met other moms with similar stories. After several months she felt like herself.

Obsessive-Compulsive Disorder (OCD)

- Up to 9 percent of new mothers have OCD.
- Of those, over 38 percent also have depression.

Symptoms May Include

- Intrusive, repetitive, and persistent thoughts or mental pictures
- Thoughts often are about hurting or killing the baby
- Tremendous sense of horror and disgust about these thoughts
- Thoughts may be accompanied by behaviors to reduce the anxiety (for example, hiding knives)
- Counting, checking, cleaning or other repetitive behaviors
- Fear of germs
- Fears about her own health

Risk Factor

Personal or family history of obsessive-compulsive disorder. (diagnosed or not)

Tanya's Story

Each time I went near the balcony I would clutch my baby tightly until I was in a room with the door closed. Only then did I know he was safe one more time from me dropping him over the edge. The bloody scenes I would envision horrified me. Passing the steak knives in the kitchen triggered images of my stabbing the baby, so I asked my husband to hide the knives. I never bathed my baby alone since I was afraid I might drown him.

Although I didn't think I would ever really hurt my baby son, I never trusted myself alone with him. I was terrified I would "snap" and actually carry out one of these scary thoughts. If my baby got sick, it would be all my fault, so I would clean and clean to make sure there were no germs. Although I had always been more careful than other people, now I would check the locks on the windows and doors many times a day.

Tanya's Treatment

After meeting with Tanya twice individually, her therapist suggested that her husband join her in the next session. Tanya needed reassurance that her husband knew she wasn't "crazy" and would never really harm the baby. She did not want to tell him the specific graphic thoughts, so she referred to them generally as "scary thoughts." After being educated, her husband's aggravation with her being "nervous all the time" subsided.

Tanya started taking an antidepressant, and soon the scary thoughts were occurring less frequently. Her therapist suggested that she wait another few weeks to join a support group, until she felt less vulnerable, to hear about the anxieties of others. In the meantime, she was given the names and numbers of a few women to connect with who had survived this disorder.

Panic Disorder

Occurs in about 10 percent of postpartum women.

Symptoms May Include

- Episodes of extreme anxiety
- Shortness of breath, chest pain, sensations of choking or smothering, dizziness
- Hot or cold flashes, trembling, rapid heartbeat, numbness or tingling sensations
- Restlessness, agitation, or irritability
- During attack the woman may fear she is going crazy, dying, or losing control
- Panic attack may wake her up

- Often no identifiable trigger for the panic
- Excessive worry or fears (including fear of more panic attacks)

Risk Factors

- Personal or family history of anxiety or panic disorder (diagnosed or not)
- Thyroid dysfunction

Chris's Story

At about three weeks postpartum I stopped leaving my house at all except for pediatrician appointments. I was afraid I might have a panic attack in the store and not be able to take care of my baby. I never knew when that wave would begin washing over me and I would "lose it." The windows had to be open all the time or else I thought I would suffocate if I had an attack.

The first time I had a panic attack I thought I was having a major heart attack. A friend drove me to the emergency room and the doctor on call told me it was only stress. He gave me some medicine but I was too afraid to take it. I went home feeling stupid, like I had made a big deal out of nothing.

Everyone told me that breastfeeding would relax me, but it did just the opposite. I never knew how much milk my baby was getting and that really worried me. Sometimes when my milk would let down I would get a panic attack. The first therapist I saw told me I must have had issues bonding with my own mother, but I knew that wasn't true and I didn't see that therapist again. On many nights I woke up in a sweat, with my heart beating so fast and hard. My head was racing with anxious thoughts about who would take care of the baby when I died. I thought I was going crazy. I was so scared.

Chris's Treatment

Chris had her first therapy appointment over the telephone since she felt she could not go outside. Her therapist talked her through taking a bit of the medication her MD prescribed, so Chris would know she had something that would help in an emergency.

Driving was too scary for her, especially in tunnels and over bridges. Her husband drove her to her next session, following a route that avoided those obstacles. Chris needed to sit near the door during the appointment just in case she felt the need to run outside for some air. She began stress management classes at a local hospital. Her therapist urged her to sleep for at least half the night, every night. Chris's husband began taking care of the baby for the first half of the night on a regular basis. Chris noticed immediately how sleep lowered her stress level. She attended an infant massage class, which also helped.

Psychosis

Psychosis is a serious illness in which a person loses touch with reality. It occurs in one to two per thousand perinatal women.

- Onset is usually within the first two weeks after the woman gives birth.
- This disorder has a 5 percent suicide and 4 percent infanticide rate.

Symptoms May Include

- Seeing, hearing, or feeling things that others do not (for example, hearing the voice of God, or the devil, or getting "secret messages" from the television)
- Delusional thinking (for example, about the infant's death, denial of birth, or the need to kill the baby)
- Mania
- Confusion
- Paranoia
- Symptoms that come and go (she may seem normal one minute, and hearing voices the next minute)

Risk Factors

- Personal or family history of psychosis, bipolar disorder, or schizophrenia (diagnosed or not)
- Previous postpartum psychotic or bipolar episode

Mike's Story

My wife, Gloria, had a great pregnancy and a long labor. We were thrilled to have our first child, a son. But within days of his birth my wife began to withdraw into her own world. She became less and less communicative and she became more and more confused and suspicious. I almost had to carry her into the therapist's office; by that time she could hardly speak or answer questions, nor write her name on the forms her therapist gave us. I was told to take her to the hospital immediately.

When we arrived at the hospital, she became fearful and then violent. She ended up in restraints. Fortunately, she responded pretty quickly to the antipsychotic medication, and was able to come home after about a week. She continued to improve.

Over time and under the doctor's guidance, Gloria was able to wean herself off her medication.

We had always wanted two kids, so we consulted with our therapist and psychiatrist. With careful planning, we now have our second child and a very different story to tell.

Gloria's Treatment

After being released from the hospital, Gloria continued therapy and saw the psychiatrist, who carefully monitored her medication. She worked to understand and process what had happened to her. Eventually she joined a postpartum support group, which was quite helpful. Since there were no other moms present in the group who had experienced a postpartum psychosis, the group leader gave her the names and numbers of women who had "been there" and who wanted to offer support.

Post-traumatic Stress Disorder (PTSD)

PTSD can occur following life-threatening or injury-producing events such as sexual abuse or assault, or traumatic childbirth. It occurs in up to 6 percent of women; rates are higher (up to 30 percent) in parents who have a child in the intensive care unit.

Symptoms May Include

- Recurrent nightmares
- Extreme anxiety
- Reliving past traumatic events (for example, sexual, physical, and emotional events, and childbirth)

Risk Factors

- Past traumatic events
- Traumatic birth
- Severe physical complication or injury related to pregnancy or childbirth
- Baby in the neonatal intensive care unit (NICU)

Jennifer's Story

During the delivery it all came flooding back. I felt terrorized and vulnerable. I thought I had already dealt with the abuse in my childhood. It seemed that all the years of therapy were a waste of time and money. I was so embarrassed for losing control during labor. I was angry that what happened to me as a kid was still affecting me after all this time.

My therapist told me the nightmares and flashbacks would go away, but I just didn't know. It was so real—like the abuse was happening again over and over. I couldn't even leave my poor husband alone with my baby. I got the sick feeling that I couldn't trust even him. I was so messed up. I thought maybe I'd never be a normal mother.

Jennifer's Treatment

Jennifer hired a postpartum doula who took care of her and the baby for two months. Having this trusted female companion with her almost everywhere she went gave Jennifer comfort. She began weekly therapy sessions and eventually joined a support group. She and her therapist agreed that she did not need medication at this point.

Bipolar Disorder I or II (sometimes referred to as Bipolar Spectrum Disorder)

Also known as manic depression, bipolar disorders are characterized by moodswings from very high (mania) or high (hypomania) to low mood (depression). There is no available data about how often this occurs. Women usually seek treatment during an episode of depression and are commonly misdiagnosed as suffering from a depressive disorder, rather than a bipolar disorder.

Symptoms

- Mania (bipolar I) or hypomania (low level of mania in bipolar II; see the appendix for a description)
- Depression
- Rapid and severe mood swings

Risk Factor

Personal or family history of bipolar disorder (diagnosed or not)

Tammy's Story

After my son was born I was happier than I'd ever been in my life. Everything felt wonderful. Everyone told me I should sleep when my baby slept, but I was too excited to sleep. I was really proud of myself that I kept the house spotless, took care of my baby, and was still able to look great. My husband was pleased that dinner would always be ready for him when he came home. I was handling everything like a supermom, and felt on top of the world. After about two weeks my world started spinning out of control. I crashed. I started crying very easily and then a minute later I hated my husband and wanted a divorce. I started doing weird things like tape recording the baby all day so I could study his cries. I would also record my thoughts since I believed they were profound and should be documented. My head would not slow down for a second. It was exhausting.

Tammy's Treatment

Unfortunately, Tammy was first misdiagnosed as having postpartum depression, and she was given an antidepressant. She became more manic. She finally found a psychiatrist who diagnosed her as having bipolar disorder. Tammy was prescribed an antipsychotic medication for a few weeks to sedate her enough to sleep at night when her husband was watching the baby. She was also put on a mood stabilizer. In therapy, she began to understand what had happened to her, and set up realistic expectations for herself as a mother and wife. She started taking omega-3 supplements. Eventually her moods became stable. When she and her husband are ready to have another baby, she will create a treatment plan with her psychiatrist for pregnancy and postpartum.

Consequences of *Untreated* Parental Depression on Children

Maternal depression was placed at the top of the list entitled "Most significant mental health issues impeding children's readiness for school" (Mental Health Policy Panel, Department of Health Services, 2002). There is a tremendous amount of data that show what a negative impact untreated maternal and paternal depression has on fetuses, babies, and other children in the home. That impact may continue through childhood and into the teen years. Fifty percent of children of depressed moms will have depression by the end of adolescence. At least 10 percent of fathers are moderately or severely depressed. Depressed fathers are nearly 4 times more likely to spank, and less than 50 percent of these dads report regularly reading to their 1-year-olds. Children of depressed parents are more likely to suffer from childhood psychiatric disturbance, behavior problems, poor social functioning, and impaired cognitive and language development. When a depressed parent goes untreated, every member of the family and all the relationships within the family are affected. The quicker the parent is treated, the better it is for the entire family. The longer the depression remains, the more likely the children and family are to suffer depression. Suicide is the second leading cause of death in new mothers during the first year.

These are very sobering statistics; however, we want to emphasize the heading of this section. It's *untreated* parental depression that causes problems. The takeaway message is, of course, get treated right away to help insure a healthy family.

Perinatal Loss

No matter how a pregnancy ends, whether by nature or by choice, depression and anxiety may follow. Not only should grief be addressed through counseling, and other types of treatment may also be useful. Although miscarriage occurs frequently (over 20 percent of pregnancies), often women don't talk about it. Many people are uncomfortable talking about death and loss, so it's important to find support and know you are not alone. Don't assume you should be depressed or anxious—get support if you feel it will help you get through this rough time. Women who have experienced any neonatal loss need to be monitored carefully for distress in future pregnancies and the postpartum period.

When there is a pregnancy loss, both parents suffer. Each person grieves differently, and counseling for the couple can be helpful. Moms go through an immediate physiological and emotional reaction. Partners often feel they need to be "strong", and the "rock" to support the mom through the grieving process. Partners are often the ones taking care of details and are on "autopilot." In a study in the United Kingdom, 36 percent of dads suffered from severe anxiety at six weeks after a pregnancy loss. Interestingly, dads were found to have more depression than the moms at thirteen months after the loss. It may be that as the mom's depression post-loss improves, the partners fall apart. This can cause tension in the relationship. Sometimes women interpret their partners' initial stoic response as a lack of caring. Couples really need to communicate to work as a team and support each other. Among other measures, the support plan should include nutrition, sleep, social support, and possible medication.

We have included some helpful references in the Resources section of this book.

Three
Women with Perinatal Disorders

This chapter is for you if you are suffering. In the chapters to follow, we will discuss the role of practitioners, partners, and other family members in helping mothers recover.

Among the women we treat are those in the healthcare and educational professions, such as MDs, nurses, daycare and preschool providers, teachers, and therapists, to name a few. We often hear from these women, "This can't be happening to me! I take care of everyone else in crisis." What we tell them is that our brain doesn't care what we do for a living! No one is immune. No matter what the educational or socioeconomic level, culture, religion, or personality, wherever women are having babies, the statistics remain consistent.

Women who suffer perinatal emotional difficulty experience their emotional pain in many different ways. Here are some of the common feelings they express:

No one has ever felt as bad as I do.
I'm all alone. No one understands.
I'm a failure as a woman, mother, and wife.
I'll never be myself again.
I've made a terrible mistake.
I'm on an emotional roller coaster.
I'm losing it.
I wasn't cut out to be a mom.

Please know that each woman may experience these feelings at varying levels. Some may feel all of them, and others may feel only a few. You might also recognize some of your symptoms listed in Chapter 2.

Finding a Therapist or Medical Practitioner

We encourage you to contact Postpartum Support International (PSI) at 800-944-4PPD (944-4773) or postpartum.net to locate a therapist who has shown interest and commitment in the postpartum field. PSI, along with other organizations, provides specialized training in perinatal mood and anxiety disorders. We have not found any graduate training that fully covers this material. Do not assume (as many insurance companies would like you to believe) that someone who has expertise in working with depression or anxiety is knowledgeable about the unique aspects of perinatal mood and anxiety disorders.

Most insurance companies have coverage for mental health. It is usually less expensive if you see a provider on their "panel." Sometimes an insurance company is willing to add a specialist to its provider list or pay for you to see one. If your insurance company will pay only if you see providers on their list, here are screening questions to help you determine their knowledge in this area. It's important to ask these questions, even if the therapist considers himself or herself knowledgeable. If you don't have the energy to deal with the insurance company or to screen professionals, ask a support person to do this for you. Medical practitioners should be asked if they are comfortable prescribing psychiatric medication (if needed) to a pregnant or breastfeeding mother.

- *What specific training have you received in perinatal mood and anxiety disorders?*

- *Do you belong to any organization dedicated to education about perinatal mood and anxiety disorders?* Someone committed to working in this field should belong to at least one of these organizations: Postpartum Support International, Marcé Society, North American Society for Psychosocial OB/GYN.

- *What books do you recommend to women with prenatal or postpartum depression or anxiety?* Someone with expertise should be able to name several books listed in the Resources section of this book.

- *What is your theoretical orientation?* Research has shown the most effective types of therapy for your condition are cognitive-behavioral and interpersonal. You are experiencing a life crisis; long-term intensive psychoanalysis is not appropriate.

If you are unable to find a therapist with expertise, interview until you find someone who is compassionate and willing to learn. If you do not think a practitioner is helping you, move on! Be a good consumer. Shop around until you feel satisfied that you are in capable hands.

The Truth of the Matter

As you face the challenge of a perinatal mood or anxiety disorder, remind yourself of these truths:

- *I will recover!*
  We have never met a woman who, after proper treatment, did not recover.

- *I am not alone!*
  One in five women will experience perinatal illness.

- *This is not my fault!*
  You did not create this; it is a real illness.

- *I am a good mom!*
  Even if you are hospitalized, you are still making sure your baby is provided for. The fact that you are trying to improve the quality of your life and your family's proves you are a good mom.

- *It is essential for me to take care of myself!*
  It is your job to take care of yourself so you can get better and take care of your family.

- *I am doing the best I can.*
  No matter what your current level of functioning, you are taking steps, regardless of how small they seem. Good for you!

Depression may interfere with your ability to believe these statements, so it is important to say them frequently, as if you really mean them. As you recover, this exercise will become easier.

Basic Mom Care

Women today are expected to be supermoms and do it all. There is a lot of pressure to have a perfect baby who never cries, a clean and well-organized home, and a happy, supportive partner. Even when there are helpful people around, many women are uncomfortable asking for help. We often hear the expression "it takes a village," but many feel that asking for or needing help is a sign of weakness. You deserve to be well no matter how much help it takes.

Finding Support People

Very often when we are in crisis, we overlook the people around us who can be of help and support. People can support you in different ways, and all types of support are needed. Physical support can be cooking, cleaning, caring for the baby, shopping, or taking you for a walk or to an appointment. Emotional support may include sitting and listening, hugging, and giving encouraging words. Accept all the help that's offered and ask for more.

This is a brainstorming exercise—write down everyone who comes to mind, regardless of the type of support he or she may be able to give you. If possible, do this exercise with a support person. Keep this list of supporters' names and phone numbers handy by your phone in times of need.

Here are some places where our clients have found support. Think about how these sources might help you the best:

- Partner
- Friends
- Family and extended family
- Neighbors
- Coworkers
- Religious communities
- Professionals (including doulas, lactation consultants, nannies, housekeepers)
- Hotlines and warmlines
- Online postpartum depression message boards (see the Resources section)
- Prenatal/Postpartum depression support groups

Do not assume that because someone is in a helping profession or is family, he or she will be helpful or understanding. Find and surround yourself with nonjudgmental, caring support.

Eating

Often women with perinatal depression and anxiety crave sweets and carbohydrates. If you can eat something nutritious, especially protein, each time you feed the baby, you can help keep your blood sugar level even. This will contribute to keeping your mood stable. We understand this may be difficult if you are experiencing a lack of appetite, so do the best you can. If you have trouble eating, try drinking your food—for example, protein shakes or drinks. Avoid caffeine.

Ask a support person to shop for things like yogurt, sliced deli meat and cheese, hardboiled eggs, precut vegetables, fruit, and nuts. Better yet, if they are not already offering, ask people to bring you food. Don't forget to drink water—dehydration can increase anxiety. Appetite problems are quite common with perinatal depression and anxiety. Please tell your health practitioner about any major appetite or weight changes. It might be helpful to consult a nutritionist who is familiar with depression and anxiety when you have the energy.

A recent study of over one thousand women looked at the effect of diet on depression and anxiety. Women (across age, socioeconomic status, education, and health habits) who ate a diet high in vegetables, fruit, meat, fish, and whole grains had less depression and anxiety. Women who ate a diet of processed or fried foods, refined grains, sugary products, and beer had higher rates of depression and anxiety.

Sleeping

Mood is severely affected by lack of sleep. Moms are more depressed, irritable, and anxious when they have interrupted sleep. Nighttime sleep is the most valuable sleep in helping you recover. Sleep is necessary to restore brain health and ideally, the brain needs eight hours of uninterrupted sleep each night. Although with only six hours of uninterrupted sleep the ability to think clearly and respond is decreased, it's often a more reasonable goal for many families with a new baby. You need to be "off duty" physically, emotionally, and psychologically for a few hours per night. The baby can be fed breast milk in a bottle or formula by your partner or other support person. You can either split each night with your partner or alternate taking a full night "on," then a full night "off."

If you don't have a partner or your partner is not home, you will need to enlist a support person to be responsible for the baby during this time. When you are "off," you should sleep away from the baby in another room, with earplugs. Many of our clients also use a fan, air purifier, or another appliance to block all baby noises.

Remember, it is your job to take care of yourself. Even if you cannot arrange for this nightly, a few nights a week will help. If you are able to nap in the day, do so, but naps do not replace nighttime sleep. Sleep problems occur frequently with mood and anxiety disorders. If you are unable to sleep at night when everyone else is sleeping, please talk to your health practitioner.

Physical Activity

Even a few minutes of brisk physical activity can help your mood. When you are physically able to be active, find something you are willing to do (for example, walking, dancing, or bike riding). If the thought of walking around the block is overwhelming, start slowly and work up. It will get easier as you feel better. If you know you would feel better if you did the activity, but it is hard to mobilize yourself, designate a support person or buddy to encourage you and participate with you. Pregnant and postpartum women who got some exercise (including walking with a stroller) were found to cope better and have a reduction in depression.

If you have sleep problems or are very sleep deprived, do not do intense aerobics—this can actually make your sleep condition worse. Wait until you have had at least a couple of weeks of good sleep before you resume or begin a heavy exercise program.

Taking Breaks

The myth is that if we really love our children enough, we shouldn't need breaks from them or have fun without them. This certainly isn't the case! We've bought into the idea that taking time for ourselves is selfish and bad, and therefore we feel guilty when we even think we need a break. There's no other job that's 24/7. The truth is that all good mothers take breaks—that's how they stay good mothers. We strongly recommend that you get regularly scheduled time off each week for a minimum of two hours at a time (this does not include chores and errands—pleasure only). For every job other than being a mother, breaks are mandated by law, and you'd expect much more time off.

If you don't recharge your batteries, you'll be running on empty. You are not the only one who can care for the baby. Partners and family members, for instance, should be given alone time to bond with the baby too. This experience is important for the baby, and it can be done more easily with you somewhere else. Everyone wins.

If you are not able to leave the house, go to another room and use earplugs or headphones. Or maybe your support person can leave the house with the baby and give you time alone.

Going Outside

When you are depressed or anxious, the four walls feel as if they're closing in. The world feels darker and smaller. You tend to fold in emotionally and physically (as in crossing your arms, hunching over, and fixing your gaze downward).

We encourage you to go outside your home, look up at the sky, stand up straight, put your arms at your sides, and breathe. You don't have to actually go anywhere. Just go outside once a day, even if this means standing outside your front door in your bathrobe.

Improving Your Mood—Take Control of Your Environment

Avoid reading or listening to the news. If you want to watch a movie, choose a comedy. Avoid tragic or violent films. Open the drapes and curtains and let the sunlight in. If you are anxious, listen to soothing music. If you are depressed, try music with a good beat that gets your body moving.

Taking Care of the Baby

Depending on the level of depression, you may need someone to do most, if not all, of the baby care. A support person, such as a family member, doula, nanny, or friend, can be with you when your partner is not. Very gradually you can increase your participation with the baby care as your support person keeps you company.

Even though you may feel like a robot at first, just going through the motions without joy, it is still good for you to experience yourself doing some "mommy" tasks and interacting with the baby. Your feelings of competence and confidence will increase, and eventually you will be able to enjoy your day. Smile, touch, and interact with your baby as much as you're able. Once you're up to it, you might find it helpful to sign up for an infant massage or baby swimming class. These types of classes promote mother-infant bonding.

Scripts

You may not know what you need when a support person asks, "What can I do?" It's all right to say, "I don't know what I need right now. I just know I feel awful." However, don't assume anyone can read your mind. You are most likely to get what you need if you ask for it.

Try giving your partner, family, and friends a script to guide them in how to best support you. For example, when you are experiencing anxiety, it will not be helpful to hear, "Just calm down and relax." Instead, try giving them suggestions of what to say and do:

I am sorry you are suffering.
We will get through this.
I am here for you.
Hug.
This will pass.

A script does not detract from the genuineness of caring and love. On the contrary, it will give your support people an effective way to give you what you need. People who love you want you to get better. They will be relieved to know what will help.

For Women with Anxiety, Fear, or Extreme Worry

Be sure to avoid caffeine and keep your blood sugar level even (see the section titled "Eating"). For many women with anxiety or obsessions, information provides fuel for worry. Turn off the TV news, and don't read the news. Don't read books, magazines, or Internet information if you find it makes you more anxious. Avoid all media—including social media—if it fuels your worry or fear. If you go to the movies, select comedies. Find activities that can soothe or distract you, rather than those that stir up anxiety.

Preventing Too Much Stimulation

When the usual sights, sounds, and daily activity feel like too much, it is important to adjust your surroundings. Remember, you are in recovery. Treating yourself with "kid gloves" can greatly boost your recovery. Don't push yourself. If, for instance, going to a family event seems overwhelming (even if you have had fun at this event in the past), you probably should not go. Trust yourself. As you recover, you'll be able to handle more.

Perinatal women often feel hypersensitive to stimulation of all kinds—visual (seeing), auditory (hearing), and kinesthetic (touch). If this is happening, it may be soothing to lower the light in your house. (If you are feeling more depressed than anxious, try brightening your house with more light—open your curtains and add lamps, for example.) As long as you can hear what you need to, try wearing earplugs or headphones during the day to muffle unnecessary noise. You may become more sensitive to touch—for instance, clothing may rub, scratch, or itch. Be compassionate with yourself and do what you need to in order to be comfortable.

Myths About Nursing

Myth: "I can't be a good mom unless I nurse my baby."

The truth is there is no one right way to feed your baby. Whatever works for you and your family is the right way. There is a tremendous amount of pressure on new moms in our society to nurse exclusively, regardless of physical or emotional obstacles. We believe that one size never fits all. Whether you feed your baby breast milk (from breast or bottle) or formula has no relationship to how much you love your child or what kind of mother you are.

There are advantages and disadvantages to both breastfeeding and bottle feeding, and some combination of the two may work for you as well. For instance, having a support person bottle feed with formula or breast milk so you can be off duty is a responsible choice for your family's well-being. Don't allow yourself to be guilt-tripped!

Be prepared for intrusive and inappropriate questions and comments about how you're feeding your baby. This may happen anywhere, for example, out in public, at your health practitioner's office, in a moms' group, or at a family gathering. If any person, whether lay or professional, seems judgmental about the plan you've chosen, remind yourself that you have made the best decision you can for you and your family. You can ignore the question or comment or change the subject. Alternatively, you can say, "It's none of your business," "I can't breastfeed. I have a life-threatening illness," "I chose not to," or "My doctor told me I can't." Women who breastfeed in public may also get comments. Be prepared.

Remember, you are entitled to respond any way you need to in order to get people off your back. You have nothing to apologize about and you do not owe them an explanation. Good moms make sure their babies are fed. Period.

Myth: "My baby won't bond if I don't nurse."

If this were true, there would be whole generations of adults who never bonded with their mothers. Some women actually begin to bond with their babies when they stop breastfeeding. For women who are experiencing anxiety or pain related to breastfeeding, bottle feeding (formula or breast milk) or a combination of breastfeeding and bottle feeding may allow this time together to be more relaxed and enjoyable. Also, there are no rules about how to bottle feed. If you desire skin-to-skin contact, you can bottle feed bare-chested. Bottle feeding provides a chance for good eye contact and connection. Just because a mom is breastfeeding, she might not be using that as a bonding opportunity. There are many chances throughout the day to bond with your baby, such as diaper changing, cuddling, bathing, smiling at your baby, and so on. Feeding is not the only time for bonding to take place. Bonding is an ongoing process of interaction, for moms as well as partners. It goes far beyond how or what you feed your baby.

Myth: "My baby can sense my depression or anxiety."

Your baby cannot read your mind. Your thoughts or feelings will not damage your baby or the relationship with your baby. What babies can sense is temperature, hunger, wetness, and physical contact. Your baby will feel close to you regardless of depressed or anxious thoughts running through your head. It's your behavior that counts (smiling, talking, touching, and so on). Having a nondepressed caretaker in charge of the baby for part of the time will also help as you recover.

Myth: "Bonding happens only immediately at birth."

No adopted children would ever bond with their adoptive parents if this were true. There is no one magic moment of opportunity when bonding must happen, and no reason to worry about bonding if you were unable to touch or hold your baby immediately after delivery. Even if your depression or anxiety has made it difficult for you to care for your baby, it's never too late. Bonding is a process of familiarity, closeness, and comfort that continues for years.

Recovery

What will help each woman recover depends on the type, severity, and unique aspects of her illness and her preferences for treatment. Whatever helps you get better quickly is what we recommend. In Chapter 7 we outline a few different treatment options that you may choose to do separately or in combination. Since medication is among the most common treatments for these disorders, we've discussed a few of the questions and concerns we hear most often.

Antidepressant Questions and Answers

Question: Will medication change my personality?

Answer: Depression and anxiety change your personality — people who are usually easygoing and stable may become irritable, moody, withdrawn, or worried. As the medication begins to work, you will begin to feel like yourself again. In a sense, medication restores you to your "old" personality.

Question: How long will I have to take the medicine?

Answer: Treatment length varies, and is a decision between you and your prescribing practitioner. If this is your first episode of depression/anxiety, the general recommendation is to take a dose that gets you "back to yourself," then continue on the medicine for a minimum of nine months to a year. If you have a history of depression or anxiety, your practitioner may suggest a longer course of treatment. Staying on the medication for the recommended time is critical to reduce your chances of having a relapse or recurrence of illness.

Question: Will I become dependent on the antidepressant?

Answer: Antidepressants are not addictive, but you should never stop taking them suddenly. Speak with your practitioner, who will guide the process of weaning yourself off the medication. Some psychiatrists recommend two to four months to taper off the antidepressant. Most women (depending upon their history of illness) are able to go off medication at some point.

Question: What if I have side effects?

Answer: Many people experience no side effects at all. If side effects do occur, they are usually mild and temporary, lasting less than a week (nausea, fatigue, or shakiness, for instance). If you experience a decrease in sex drive or ability to orgasm, it may persist through the course of treatment. If you feel more severe side effects or side effects that do not clear up after a week, contact your practitioner. Some women need to try more than one antidepressant before they find the one that works best for them. To reduce the likelihood of side effects, it is helpful to start at a very low dose and slowly work up to the dosage that is effective for you.

Question: Which antidepressant is the right one for me?

Answer: In general, most people do well on most of the antidepressant medications. If you have previously been on a medication that was helpful, or if you have a blood relative doing well on a medication, that one would probably be the first choice. If you are anxious, a medication that may have a calming side effect might be chosen. If you have fatigue, a medication that may have an energizing side effect may be tried. The most important indicator is whether you begin to feel better over time.

Question: When will I feel better? How will I know if the medication is working?

Answer: Most of the newer antidepressants begin working within two weeks, while the older medications can take four to six weeks to work. Here are some comments we have heard as the medicine begins working:

- I'm not crying all the time.
- I have more patience—my fuse is longer.
- I'm singing in the shower again.
- My husband noticed I seem happier.
- I feel more motivated—I'm cooking for the family again.
- I'm enjoying the baby more.
- I'm not worrying as much—the little things aren't getting to me.
- I'm smiling and laughing more, and having fun.
- I'm answering email and phone calls again.

Question: Won't medication be a crutch?

Answer: A crutch is a temporary tool that you use until you no longer need it. If you broke your foot you wouldn't think twice about using crutches to support you while your foot heals. Medication restores your brain chemistry to a normal state, allowing you to get back to feeling yourself and back to your life. As you become well, you and your doctor will develop a plan to wean you off the medication. Additionally, medication can help you utilize psychotherapy more effectively.

Question: I want to breastfeed, but I don't want to take anything that will harm my baby. Can I take medication and nurse?

Answer: According to the professionals who have dedicated their careers to studying the safety of antidepressants and nursing, the answer is yes. When infant blood was examined, few, if any, metabolites of medication were found. Babies exposed to medication through breast milk are as healthy and normal in all ways as babies not exposed to medication. It's always important to remember that going untreated can affect the baby's health and is not a good option.

It's clear from the research that it is more important for a mom to receive proper treatment than whether she feeds her baby breast milk or formula. So if you think you will worry too much about your baby if you continue using breast milk while taking an antidepressant, it is better to wean yourself (slowly) rather than to go without treatment. Remember that the best gift you can give your baby is a happy, healthy mom. Often the fear about using breast milk while taking a medication goes away once the medication starts working, since the worry can be caused by the illness itself.

Question: I am pregnant and really depressed. Do I need to feel this way for the rest of my pregnancy?

Answer: About 15 to 23 percent of women experience depression in pregnancy. Getting treatment is important for both you and the baby. Researchers have begun looking at the harmful effects of untreated depression and anxiety on the fetus. Also, if you are depressed or anxious in pregnancy, you may not be caring for yourself as you need to. This is not good for you or your developing baby. Many women are tempted to self-medicate, for example with caffeine, cigarettes, alcohol, drugs, or herbs, and this too can be harmful.

Counseling alone may be enough, but for some, medication is necessary to reduce serious symptoms. Antidepressants have been shown to be helpful for both depression and anxiety. No increased risk of miscarriage or malformations has been shown to result from taking these medications, even in the first trimester. Depression in pregnancy also puts you at high risk for postpartum depression, and can put the baby at risk for developmental delays. Being on medication through pregnancy and postpartum will significantly decrease this risk.

Question: I am embarrassed and ashamed about taking medication. Am I weak because I need a medication?

Answer: There is a stigma in our culture about people who take psychiatric medication. This stigma is based on ignorance. Somehow it is presumed we can control our brain chemistry. If you had diabetes or a thyroid disorder you wouldn't expect (and no one would suggest) that you could will yourself to make more insulin or thyroid hormone. It's a strength to get help when we need it, not a weakness.

Taking medication is a personal choice. You are not required to share this information with others. Being private is not the same as being ashamed. However, once our clients begin to tell close family or friends, they are often surprised to find out how many of them are also on medication, or know someone who is. Whether you choose to take an antidepressant or not, find people who will support your choices for wellness.

Four
Partners

This chapter is designed to provide support to you, the partner, regardless of your gender or marital status. To avoid confusion, we sometimes refer to the new mother as "wife." The sooner you become involved in the recovery process, and the greater your involvement, the more you both will benefit—together and separately. The more you understand what she is experiencing, the better supported she will feel. That will, in turn, speed her recovery.

Having a baby brings changes to the whole family. Questions like, "Will I be a good parent?" and "How can I best support my partner through this uncharted territory?" are normal and healthy to ask. This happens in all types of relationships—heterosexual, gay and lesbian couples, and adoptive parents. Having a baby changes things. Attention that had gone to the dad or partner now goes to the pregnancy. Fears, discomfort, and medical problems can affect intimacy. Once the baby is born, attention goes to the baby, and the couple relationship is on the back burner. We hear more these days about women's mood problems during pregnancy and postpartum, but we hear very little mentioned about the mental health of dads and partners. Dads and partners are important, too!

Most often we are told the glowing side of parenthood; you will feel instantly bonded and fall madly in love. That may happen, but often it's a process of getting to know this demanding stranger. There are losses associated with becoming a parent, and it's important to acknowledge and grieve them. It is normal for your relationship with your partner to change. If she's (or you've) been drooled on, spit up on, and sucked on all day, she (or you) may be "touched out." It's easy to feel rejected. Remind yourself, it's not a personal rejection. You can no longer jump into bed, take off to the movies, or go out to dinner on a whim.

It is now thought that about 15 to 23 percent of women suffer from mood or anxiety problems during pregnancy. Some women go into pregnancy with a past or current history, and others develop a new onset of an illness. And, as many as one in five women will have a postpartum mood or anxiety disorder.

Likewise, some dads or partners may have a history of, or may be experiencing, a mood or anxiety disorder during the pregnancy. Depression and anxiety disorders (in particular obsessive-compulsive disorder) worsen during times of stress and sleep deprivation. It's important for dads to assess their own risk going into a pregnancy.

What do depressed or anxious dads look like? They look like dads. You can't tell by looking. When a mother is experiencing a prenatal or postpartum mood or anxiety disorder, her partner is at an increased risk of suffering as well. In a study published in 2006, 10 percent of fathers showed moderate to severe depression nine months after the birth of a baby. Another study found that paternal mood and anxiety disorders in the first two months postpartum occurred in up to 25 percent of dads. Two more recent studies (2009 and 2010) found rates of 10 percent of postpartum depression in dads. The highest rates were seen three to six months postpartum. When the mom is depressed, the rate of depression in her partner is significantly higher—24 to 50 percent. If the partner has a history of depression or anxiety, this is a high risk factor with or without depression in the mom. We suggest that all new moms and partners be screened on a routine basis.

Not all depressed men or women experience extreme sadness. Often, especially in men, depression may be seen as irritability, aggression, and hostility. They may distance themselves, find distractions to avoid the family, or "check out." This certainly contributes to relationship or marital distress. Other common symptoms may be difficulty falling or staying asleep, appetite changes, racing thoughts or constant worry, lack of joy or pleasure in things that used to be enjoyed. Some people feel helpless and hopeless. Having a new baby and an increased financial burden can really contribute to a feeling of being trapped. Being depressed is like having dark glasses on. Everything you see gets filtered through the lenses and gets distorted. Only the negative things get though.

Depression in dads also affects childhood behavioral and emotional development. Children 3.5 years old were found to have problems, boys more than girls. Four-year-old children of fathers with major depression were more likely to have been treated by professionals for speech, language, and behavioral problems. Depression in fathers is significantly associated with psychiatric disorders in their children seven years later, in particular, oppositional defiant/conduct disorders in boys.

What can dads do? Get support! Get educated! Find a professional. Talk to your partner, friends, or family, if you think they will listen. It is critical to find nonjudgmental support. Getting the help you need is a sign of strength.

To find a number of websites devoted to dad support, see the Resources section.

Things to Keep in Mind

- *You didn't cause her illness and you can't take it away.*
  Perinatal depression and anxiety are diagnosable disorders. It is no one's fault. When her brain chemistry returns to normal, she will feel like herself again. It is your job to support her as this happens.

- *She doesn't expect you to "fix it.*
  "Many partners feel frustrated because they feel inadequate or unable to fix the problem. She doesn't need you to try to take the problem away. This isn't like a leaky faucet that can be repaired with a new washer. Don't suggest quick-fix solutions. This isn't that kind of problem. She just needs you to listen.

- Get *the support you need so you can be there for her.*
  We frequently see the partner becoming depressed during or after his wife's illness. You can avoid this by taking care of yourself and getting your own support from friends, family,

or professionals. You should make sure to get breaks from taking care of your family. Regular exercise or other stress-reducing activity is important so you can remain the solid support for your wife. Provide a stand-in support person for her while you're gone. About 10 percent of postpartum dads get moderately to severely depressed. If the mom is depressed, the chances increase to 24 to 50 percent.

- *Don't take it personally.*
  Irritability is common with perinatal depression/anxiety. Don't allow yourself to become a verbal punching bag. It's not good for anyone concerned. She feels guilty after saying hurtful things to you. If you feel you didn't deserve to be snapped at, explain that to her calmly.

- *Just being there with and for her is doing a great deal.*
  Being present and letting her know you support her is often all she'll need. Ask her what words she needs to hear for reassurance, and say them to her often.

- *Have realistic expectations.*
  Even a non-depressed postpartum woman cannot realistically be expected to cook dinner, clean house, and care for the baby. She might feel guilty about not measuring up to her own expectations and worry that you will also be disappointed. Remind her that parenting your child and taking care of your home is also your job, not just hers. Your relationship and family will emerge from this crisis stronger than ever. Very often there will be good days and bad days. Gradually, the frequency and severity of bad days will decrease. Don't assume, though, that after a few good days she is "cured." It may be a number of months before she is consistently having good days.

- *Let her sleep at night.*
  She needs at least six hours of uninterrupted sleep per night for brain health. If you want your wife back quicker, be on duty during this time without disturbing her. Many dads

and partners have expressed how much closer they are to their children because of nighttime caretaking. If you can't be up with the baby during the night, hire someone who can take your place. A temporary baby nurse will be worth his or her weight in gold.

- *Be on her team.*
  Help her figure out if her plan is working. Tell her when you see improvement like, "You're smiling more" or "You're calling your friends again." If you don't see her improving over time, gently let her know your concerns and offer to accompany her to her next appointment.

What to Say, What Not to Say

Say:

- *We will get through this.*
- *I'm here for you.*
- *I'm on your team.*
- *I won't leave you—we're here for each other through thick and thin.*
- *I know you'll get well.*
- *If there is something I can do to help you, please tell me.*
  For example, care for the baby, run her a warm bath, or put on soothing music.
- *I'm sorry you're suffering. That must feel awful.*
- *I love you very much.*
- *The baby loves you very much.*
- *This is temporary.*
- *You'll get yourself back.*
  As she recovers, point out specifics about how you see her old self returning, such as smiling again, having more patience, or going out with her friends.
- *You're doing such a good job.*
  Give specific examples.

- *You're a great mom.*
  Give specific examples, such as "I love how you smile at the baby."

- *This isn't your fault. If I were ill, you wouldn't blame me, and you'd take care of me.*

Do Not Say:

- *Think about everything you have to feel happy about.*
  She already knows everything she has to feel happy about. One of the reasons she feels so guilty is that she is depressed despite these things. That's the nature of depression.

- *Just relax.*
  This suggestion usually produces the opposite effect. She is already frustrated at not being able to relax despite all the coping mechanisms that have worked in the past. Anxiety produces hormones that can cause physical reactions, such as an increased heart rate, shakiness, visual changes, shortness of breath, and muscle tension. This is not something she can just will away.

- *Snap out of it.*
  If she could, she would have already. She wouldn't wish this on anyone. A person cannot snap out of any illness.

- *Just think positively.*
  It would be lovely if recovery were that simple! The nature of this illness prevents positive thinking. Depression feels like wearing foggy dark, distorted lenses that filter out positive input from the environment. Only negative, guilt-ridden interpretations of the world are perceived. This illness is keeping her from experiencing the lighter, humorous, and joyful aspects of life.

From a Dad Who's Been There

This was written by Henry, Shoshana's husband, for Shoshana's newsletter, soon after her first depression had subsided:

You've just come home from a long day at work, hoping to find a happy home—and what you find makes you want to get back into the car and leave. Your wife is in tears, the baby is crying. The house is a mess, and forget about dinner. By now you know better than to ask how her day was. Her response is always the same. "I hate this 'mother' stuff. I don't want to be anyone's mother. I want my old life back. I want to be happy again." You shrug, go to hold the baby, and wonder why your wife is feeling this way, why she's not as happy as you are about the baby, and when she will snap out of it.

You're not alone. I lived with this scene every day for two years. Every ounce of my patience was tested, but I kept hoping that things would be "normal" again. I focused on my baby daughter, the one in the midst of this mess, and kept telling myself I'd be there for her.

Slowly, slowly, my wife recovered from the illness. Today, we have that happy home we both always wanted. Be patient and tolerant. Remember, it will get better.

Five
Siblings, Family, and Friends

It's painful to watch someone you love struggle or suffer. It is often confusing and difficult to understand the illness or process of recovery. Perinatal mood and anxiety disorders are real and can be debilitating. The more educated you become, the more supportive and helpful you can be. This chapter is to support and educate you, and help you become part of the healing process.

After the birth of a baby there are many changes that occur in a household. Although older children may expect some of these changes, they probably will not be expecting Mom to be different. Even siblings who are too young to understand the concepts of depression and anxiety will most likely notice that their mother's behavior has not been normal.

Children usually notice if Mom is, or has been, crying. They will notice if Mom yells or gets angry over little things. Perhaps they will notice that Mom stays in bed more, does not have the energy to take them to the park, or does not seem to laugh much lately. Maybe they see her staring blankly into space, not paying much attention to them. Children can tell this is not the Mom they used to know, and they need honest, clear explanations about what is occurring.

It is crucial that the path of communication with children is open. Whenever possible the mother herself should talk with her children. The partner or another adult can help to reinforce the information. There are several important guidelines in communicating with children about what is happening.

Communicating with Children

- Even adults are often unclear about words like *depression* or *anxiety*. Instead, use descriptive words like *sad, cranky, tired, weepy, worried,* or *grouchy*.

51

- Reassure children often that they did not cause Mommy's illness or problem; this is not their fault, nor could they have done anything to prevent it.

- Let them know it is not the kind of illness caused by germs. She did not catch it from anyone, nor can she pass it on to them.

- Let the children know that Mom is getting help—seeing a doctor or counselor, taking medicine—and she will get better soon. Let them know Mom may have some good and some bad times as she recovers.

- Ask the children how they can help Mom. Perhaps they can draw a pretty picture, leave "I love you" notes around the house for her, and offer to help with age-appropriate tasks.

- Tell the truth. Children know if Mom is not "herself," so don't tell them she is fine when she is not. Mom should be direct and honest too. For instance, when it is apparent that she is feeling sad, she can say so. Sadness is just a feeling; it does not have to be logical or rational. Feelings are part of being human. To hide sadness (for example, saying, "Oh, these are 'happy tears"), gives the message that it is not okay to be sad.

What you can teach your children by showing feelings is how to express yourself in appropriate ways. This will not damage them. On the contrary, it can model behavior that will serve them well in the future. And by getting help you teach your children that when there is something wrong, you can do something about it.

Here is an example of what a mother could say to her child/ children:

You may have noticed I have been crying and getting mad a lot lately. Some of the chemicals in my body are not working right, and it has been affecting how I feel and how I act. I want you to know I love you very much, and I love the baby, too. I also want you to know that this is not your or anybody else's fault. I am taking good care of myself and getting help so I can get better as fast as I can. I am probably going to have good times and bad times, but I will get better and better until I'm completely well. I am looking forward to taking you to the park again. I love you very much.

Whether family and friends are related by blood or marriage, their reaction to the new mother's depression can critically affect her recovery.

Sometimes a depressed or anxious mother feels too scared to tell her partner about uncomfortable feelings, fearing disapproval and rejection. This mom may open up to you first, if given an opportunity. But even if she is talking openly with her partner, having the right kinds of support from her parents, in-laws, grandparents, siblings, and friends will provide her with the best environment for recovery.

When women become mothers, even if they aren't depressed, they often crave the company and approval of their own mothers. If a woman's own mother is deceased, or if their relationship is strained, it will be extra important to have another woman who can help fill that void. Because depressed mothers are, in general, even more vulnerable than nondepressed mothers, they will need extra reassurance from those around them, especially from adult females.

New moms in general are sensitive to criticism. Moms with perinatal mood and anxiety disorders are typically even more sensitive. Compliment the new mom frequently on her mothering and avoid negative comments, especially those related to her parenting.

Things to Keep in Mind

You will not be able to cure her.

You may feel frustrated that perinatal illnesses cannot be cured in the same way as other conditions. The course of this illness, even with medication, is different from that of an ear infection, for example. Where most common conditions get steadily better until they disappear, recovery during this time can be up and down.

Typically the woman advances two steps forward and feels better, and then drops one step back and "dips." She may feel hopeless when these dips occur, since depression robs her of a perspective that she is getting well. She may voice that she is back to square one and that she is not getting better.

It is important that you remind her that the dip is only temporary, she is getting better, and her moods will get back on track. A dip is not a step backward—it is simply part of the process. Over time the dips are shorter and not as deep, and the good times increase. Remind her that as long as she is going in the right direction overall, that is what is most important.

Encourage, do not insist.

Women suffering from these illnesses often feel incapable of finding the words to communicate their feelings. While it is positive to encourage her to share her thoughts, it is unhelpful to demand it. Let her know you are willing to listen without judging her. Trust that she will open up when she is ready and feels what she has to say will be treated seriously and respectfully. Even just being there in total silence together can be a great support. Your presence alone is tremendously helpful, even if she cannot or chooses not to speak.

Stay in the here and now.

With her up-and-down moods, the recovering woman cannot trust that the good times will last. She never knows when her moods will shift. She may be reluctant to share the good times with you for fear that you'll think she no longer needs your support. Eventually the good times will last and the dips will go away, but this process can take several weeks or even months. Reassure her that you understand she will be riding some waves in mood for a while, and that your support won't be suddenly yanked away before she's ready.

Don't let looks fool you.

Perinatal mood and anxiety disorders are often hidden illnesses. Women often appear normal to the outside world. They can look "put together," complete with makeup, jewelry, and even a smile, and be deeply depressed or anxious at the same time.

Sometimes the more depressed or anxious a mom feels, the more she overcompensates for it on the outside. For instance, if she feels ashamed, she may try to act perky in order to hide her true feelings. It is important to ask the mother how she is doing and never assume based on how she appears. So if you hear another family member say, "But she doesn't look depressed," you can teach them that looks can be quite deceiving when it comes to perinatal illness.

What to Say, What Not to Say

Say:

- *I'm here for you.*
- *I'm sorry you are suffering. That must feel awful.*
- *You're doing a great job.*
- *Be specific whenever you can.*
  "You're a great mom. I love how you smile at the baby."
- *You're a great...(sister, daughter, aunt).*
- *You will get well.*
- *Would you like me to do...(insert task)*
- *I went through this, too.*
  Only if you truly did—remember, this is not just "Baby Blues" and will not go away in a few days. If it's not true, don't say it.

Do Not Say:

- *Just buck up and tough it out.*
  Not getting adequate treatment puts women at risk of chronic illness and relapse.
- *I don't get what the big deal is.*
  Depression makes everything feel like a big deal. She's overwhelmed and unable to cope. Even small chores may seem too difficult.

- *You have so much to be happy about.*
  She knows that already. She feels guilty that she is still depressed despite those things. Depression makes it hard to see the positive.

- *You just need more sleep.*
  Sleep is important, but is usually not all she needs to be well.

- *You just need a break from your baby.*
  Breaks are crucial, but usually they are not all that is needed.

- *I went through this too.*
  This is not just "Baby Blues." Don't minimize her experience by saying you've "been there" unless you really have suffered with this illness.

- *Women have been having babies for centuries.*
  And a certain percentage has been getting depressed for centuries!

What You Can Do to Help

- Make dinner.
- Watch the baby (or her other children) so she can take a break.
- Do the laundry.
- Do the dishes.
- Make lunch for her.
- Sit and listen.
- Clean the house.
- Take a walk together.
- Go shopping or do errands for her.
- Write thank you notes for her.
- If her partner is not home, be on duty at night so she can sleep.

Six
Health Practitioners

All providers who touch the lives of pregnant and postpartum women need this information. The fact that you are reading this book clearly indicates that you are a caring and concerned professional. Your guidance during this critical time will significantly impact the mental and physical well-being of women with perinatal mood disorders. It is important not to underreact or overreact to these women's symptoms. Just treat them as matter-of-factly as you would any other common perinatal experience, for example, gestational diabetes.

This chapter contains answers to the questions that we have been asked most frequently throughout the years regarding signs, symptoms, and treatment. Because a distressed woman's contact with a professional office includes the receptionist and nursing staff, it is imperative that the entire staff be knowledgeable about the information in this book. We have created sections for primary care providers (family practitioners, internists, osteopaths, chiropractors), pediatricians, OB/GYNs and midwives, psychiatrists, birth doulas, postpartum doulas and visiting nurses, lactation consultants, childbirth educators, new parent group leaders, and adjunct professionals.

Please remember that warning signs of distress are not always obvious for a variety of reasons. Shame, guilt, or fear of judgment may cause the woman to hide her feelings. She may present more "socially acceptable" complaints such as fatigue, headache, marital problems, or a fussy baby. Just because a woman is smiling or well groomed, don't assume that she feels good. These are hidden illnesses. Although there are risk factors to help predict PMADs, there is no particular "type" of person who becomes ill. Studies have shown that standardized screening improves detection (see "Screening" section for more information).

We appreciate that you may be apprehensive about asking questions that could open a Pandora's box. She might feel accused of being a bad mom, and become defensive. But once she hears your matter-of-fact tone, and understands no shame should be attached to issues of mental health, she will be able to accept the information. She'll "get" that the brain is part of the body that deserves help when needed. In the long run, you will be saving yourself time while providing quality care.

Culture and Language

Although the prevalence of perinatal mood and anxiety disorders appears to be generally the same throughout the world, reactions to these disorders vary among cultures. Where shame is a great personal threat, for example, women may be more reluctant to discuss their symptoms and will require considerable reassurance.

Those assisting women with these disorders should take into account that nonverbal communication varies among cultures as well. For instance, a nod could signify understanding or simply respect for authority. It is also important to make clear what your role is in order to avoid unrealistic expectations.

Sociocultural factors and literacy levels should be considered when taking a history or completing an assessment. The perception of stress and types of stressors, as well as coping styles, differ across cultures. These will affect the woman's response to recommendations regarding which treatment methods to use or to avoid.

The level of simplicity or sophistication you use should be attuned to that of the patient, but do not assume that an educated woman will automatically understand her condition better than a woman with less education. For instance, avoid raising questions of self-diagnosis, such as, "Do you think you have postpartum depression?" even when a patient is highly educated. She may have a preconceived idea of what that term means. Instead, ask specific questions about her mood and behavior, which will elicit this information. These questions are outlined later in this chapter.

What to Say, What Not to Say

Say:

- *These feelings are quite common.*
- *This is treatable.*
- *You will get well*
- *Here is some information that will help you.*

Do Not Say:

- *This is normal.*
  Depression and anxiety, while common, are not normal.

- *Join a new moms' group.*
  If a mother is clinically depressed or anxious, this may be a damaging suggestion, depending largely on the leader of the group. A depressed mother is already feeling different and inadequate compared to other new mothers. Attending a "normal" new-mothers' group may intensify her alienation.

  If you know that the leader of the group is sensitive (such as those reading this book) and discusses mood problems, this mom will be fine in such a group. Ideally, she should join a group specifically designed for mothers with postpartum depression and anxiety. Many of our clients belong to both types of groups: one to discuss the normal new mom stuff and the other to openly express more difficult feelings.

- *Take a vacation.*
  Although a change of scenery may be nice, the depressed mother takes her brain chemistry with her. Her anxiety and depression level may actually increase due to the financial investment, leaving her baby, and guilt that the trip did not "cure" her.

- *Just get some exercise.*
  Most mothers are feeling overwhelmed. Some have barely enough energy to wash a bottle or take a shower, let alone go to the gym. Exercise alone will not cure her depression.

When she's able to leave her house and take a short walk, encourage her to do so. But, until then, this is just another setup for failure.

- *Do something nice for yourself.*
  This is always a good thing, but again, it will not be enough to regulate the depressed mother's neurotransmitters. This suggestion should be used only as part of a much larger treatment plan, not presented as a quick fix.

- *Sleep when the baby sleeps.*
  Even a nondepressed mother may have difficulty sleeping when the baby naps during the day. Especially for those mothers with high levels of anxiety, this will be impossible. What is most important is that she sleeps at night when her baby sleeps.

Screening

We recommend using standardized screening surveys specifically designed for perinatal use, such as the Postpartum Depression Screening Scale (PPDS) and Edinburgh Postnatal Depression Scale (EPDS). More general depression screens are also used including the Patient Health Questionnaire (PHQ-9), which has been validated for perinatal use. The PHQ-9 is being more widely used, and many healthcare providers are familiar with it. For your immediate use, we have outlined informal screening tools. We use the term *perinatal psychotherapist* to indicate a psychotherapist who specializes in the field of perinatal mood and anxiety disorders.

Prenatal Screening

Several prenatal screening inventories have been developed. They are listed in the Resources section. If time is too limited to use screening questionnaires, the questions in the Prepregnancy and Pregnancy Risk Assessment should be asked. At the bare minimum, the questions associated with the highest measure of risk, noted with an asterisk (*), must be asked. These are the questions relating to personal/family history of mental illness, previous postpartum mood disorder, and severe premenstrual mood changes.

Prenatal screening using the Edinburgh Postnatal Depression Scale or the PHQ-9 has been found to effectively identify women having symptoms of prenatal depression and anxiety. These symptoms require treatment and put a woman at higher risk for a postpartum mood or anxiety disorder.

Prepregnancy and Pregnancy Risk Assessment

Warning Signs

- Missed appointments
- Excessive worrying (about her own health or the health of the fetus)
- Looking unusually tired
- Crying
- Significant weight gain or loss
- Physical complaints with no apparent cause
- Flashbacks, fear, or nightmares regarding previous trauma
- Her concern that she won't be a good mother

Questions to Ask

Note: Even if your clients/patients have experienced these disorders, they may not be aware of this fact if they were never formally diagnosed. You may need to ask about their experience with the symptoms of the disorders as opposed to using diagnostic terms in order to adequately assess.

If a woman answers yes to any of the questions below, she is at an increased risk of a perinatal mood or anxiety disorder.

Have you ever had episodes of being down or sad, extreme worry, panic attacks, repetitive thoughts or behaviors that are troublesome, bipolar or extreme mood swings, loss of touch with reality, or an eating disorder?

Women with a personal history of mood or anxiety disorders need to be educated about their high risk for a perinatal episode. They should be referred to a perinatal psychotherapist to help them develop a plan of action to minimize their risk. Those women with a history of bipolar disorder or psychosis should also be referred to a psychiatrist for medication evaluation and observation during pregnancy and postpartum.

Are you taking any medications (prescription or nonprescription) or herbs on a regular basis?

Women who are self-medicating for insomnia, anxiety, sadness, or other symptoms that may indicate a mood disorder should be evaluated by a perinatal psychotherapist. Some women use caffeine, cigarettes, marijuana, herbs, alcohol, and drugs to ease emotional pain.

Have you had a previous pregnancy or postpartum mood or anxiety disorder?

Women answering yes to this question are at extremely high risk for another perinatal mood disorder. They should be referred to a perinatal psychotherapist who can help them develop a plan of action to prevent or at least minimize another occurrence.

Have you ever taken any medication for depression or anxiety or mood?

If yes, educate them about their risk of developing a perinatal mood or anxiety disorder. Observe them carefully during pregnancy and postpartum. If they are currently symptomatic, a referral to or consultation with a perinatal psychiatrist may be appropriate.

Have you ever had severe premenstrual mood changes (PMS or PMDD)?

Women whose moods are affected by hormone changes are clearly at high risk during pregnancy and postpartum since there are dramatic hormonal shifts. Educate them about their risk, and observe them carefully during pregnancy and postpartum.

Do you have any family history of mental illness (undiagnosed or diagnosed), psychiatric hospitalization or suicide?

If yes, educate them about their risk, and observe them during pregnancy and postpartum.

- Do you have any personal or family history of substance abuse?

- If pregnant, how have you been feeling physically and emotionally?

- Do you feel you have adequate emotional and physical support?

- Have you had a pregnancy or birth-related trauma (or other emotional, sexual, or physical abuse)?

- Are you experiencing any major life stressors (for example, moving, job change, deaths, financial problems)?

- Have there been any health problems for you or the fetus? Having twins, triplets, or multiple births puts the mother at an increased risk of postpartum depression.

- Do you have a personal or family history of thyroid disorder?

Postpartum Screening

A number of postpartum depression screening inventories are available. Most of them can easily be completed in a waiting room either electronically or in person. They can also be completed by phone.

The Edinburgh Postnatal Depression Screening Scale (EPDS) was developed in 1987 in Britain, by Dr. John Cox, et al. It is a ten-question self-report screening tool. It has been translated into many languages and is used all over the world. It has also been effective with teens and dads. It can be found on many Internet sites. This tool also comes in a shortened three-question version.

More recently in 2002 Dr. Cheryl Beck developed the Postpartum Depression Screening Scale (PDSS). It has been found to accurately screen for both postpartum depression and anxiety. The PDSS can be administered in either a short or long format. The total score can be broken down into seven symptom content scales when the long format is used. An elevated score in a particular symptom area indicates a greater amount of distress than average. The symptom scales are Sleeping/Eating Disturbances, Anxiety/Insecurity, Emotional Lability (mood swings), Mental Confusion, Loss of Self, Guilt/Shame, and Suicidal Thoughts.

PDSS has higher combinations of specificity and sensitivity than the EPDS in screening for major postpartum depression. Additionally, the PDSS was more likely to identify women with symptoms of sleep disturbance, mental confusion, and anxiety. If you have assessed that a woman has a postpartum mood or anxiety disorder, refer her to a perinatal specialist.

The Patient Health Questionaire-9 (PHQ9), while originally designed for use in family practice medicine to screen for depression, is being more widely used in perinatal settings.

Postpartum Risk Assessment

With your postpartum patients who were not screened prenatally, ask the first six questions from the Prepregnancy and Pregnancy Risk Assessment (the questions marked with *), as well as the Postpartum Risk Assessment.

Warning Signs in the Mother

- Missed appointments
- Excessive worrying (often about the mothers own health or the health of the baby)
- Looking unusually tired
- Requiring a support person to accompany her to appointments
- Significant weight gain or loss
- Physical complaints with no apparent cause
- Poor milk production or breastfeeding problems (could indicate thyroid dysfunction)
- Evading questions about her own well-being
- Crying
- Not willing to hold the baby or unusual discomfort handling or responding to the baby

- Not willing to allow others to care for the baby
- Excessive concern about the baby despite reassurance (for example, eating sufficiently, development, weight gain)
- Rigidity or obsessiveness (for example, regarding the baby's feeding or sleeping schedules)
- Excessive concern about appearance of herself or the baby
- Expressing that the baby doesn't like her or that she's not a good mother
- Expressing lack of partner support

Warning Signs in the Baby

- Excessive weight gain or loss
- Delayed cognitive or language development
- Decreased responsiveness to the mother

Questions to Ask

- *How are you doing?*
  Have good eye contact with her while you ask this question.

- *How are you feeling about being a mom?*
  Women who feel like they're doing a bad job or who generally don't like the job may be depressed.

- *Do you have any particular concerns?*

- *How are you sleeping (quality and quantity)?*
  Six hours of uninterrupted sleep per night are required for clear thinking and functioning.

- *Can you fall asleep and stay asleep at night when everyone else is asleep?*
  Sleep problems are common in every mood and anxiety disorder.

- *How is the baby sleeping?*
  Poor infant sleep is associated with maternal depression and anxiety.

- *Who gets up at night with the baby?*

- *Have you had any unusual or scary thoughts?*
  If yes, refer her to a perinatal psychotherapist or psychiatrist for immediate evaluation. Some thoughts may be normal; however, others many indicate obsessive-compulsive disorder (less urgent) or psychosis (emergency).

- *Are you receiving adequate physical and emotional help?*
  A good support system of family and friends can make a significant difference.

- *Do you generally feel like yourself?*
  Women with perinatal mood disorders often report not feeling like their usual selves, or having a different personality.

- *How is your appetite?*
  A significant change in appetite is a warning sign. Check for rapid weight loss or gain.

- *What and how often are you eating and drinking?*
  See the section on eating in Chapter 3.

- *If breastfeeding or pumping how is it going?*
  Poor milk production may indicate a thyroid dysfunction or be a result of anxiety.

- *If using formula, when and how quickly did you wean the baby?*
  Abrupt weaning can precipitate a mood disorder or anxiety disorder.

- *When was your last period?*
  First menses after delivery can be a precipitating factor.

- *Are you taking any medications or herbs on a regular basis?*
  Women who are self-treating for insomnia, anxiety, sadness, fatigue, or other symptoms that may indicate a mood or anxiety disorder should be evaluated by a perinatal psychotherapist.

- *Are you feeling moodier than normal (tearful, irritable, or worried)?*
  This is common in mood disorders. Refer to Chapter 2 for a more complete list of symptoms.

- *Have there been any health problems for you or the baby?*
  These factors increase the risk for mood and anxiety disorders.

- *How are you feeling toward your baby?*
  Ambivalence and anger are two examples of feelings that may indicate postpartum depression. Discomfort around the baby may indicate anxiety or OCD.

Psychotherapists, Psychologists, Social Workers

As a mental healthcare provider you may have had a relationship with the woman or couple before a pregnancy. You are a critical element in creating and being a part of her preconception planning and perinatal safety net. It is essential that you are familiar with risk factors and the most current information on how to reduce risk factors. Be familiar with the research regarding relapse and current medication recommendations for perinatal women. You can help her monitor symptoms and work with her healthcare providers. Have the information in the Resources section available for her and her providers.

Primary Care Providers

As a primary care provider, you may have a longstanding relationship with your patient. You have a good sense of her mental and physical health history. This puts you in an advantageous position to evaluate her pre-pregnancy risk, and provide appropriate direction. Your office may provide a safe haven should a mental health problem arise. Please have information from the Resources section available, as well as referrals to local professionals trained in perinatal mood and anxiety disorders.

A woman taking psychotropic medications who is pregnant or planning a pregnancy should be encouraged to consult a psychiatrist specializing in perinatal disorders in order to determine whether to continue medication. Recommendations will differ based on each woman's history. Women on medication for a bipolar disorder or psychosis should definitely be referred to a perinatal psychiatrist to develop a medication plan. These women need careful monitoring throughout pregnancy and postpartum.

Pediatricians and Neonatologists

Parents seek your advice for their children's well-being in all areas. Your words are powerful. While the focus of the pediatric visit is the baby, it is well documented that the mental health of the parents has a tremendous impact on the development of the children in the home. If the mom has been on medication during pregnancy, whenever possible, reassure the parents that the baby is fine and not experiencing any withdrawal or neonatal complications. Support the mom if she wishes to feed her baby breast milk while taking an antidepressant. It's been shown that mothers with depression or anxiety nurse or pump for shorter durations. They give up. Mothers on medication feed their babies breast milk for a longer duration then than those untreated.

Parents with babies in intensive care are at high risk for depression and anxiety. They need extra support and screening. Have referrals to local professionals trained in perinatal mood and anxiety disorders and information in the Resources section available.

We recommend you use a standardized postpartum screening tool. Women should be assessed throughout the first year. If your last visit with her is before one year postpartum, make sure she has referral information in case she needs it later.

Women already on medication, or those who you assess need a medical evaluation, should be referred to a psychiatrist specializing in perinatal mood and anxiety disorders. Screening should occur at well child visits throughout the child's first year.

OB/GYNs, Midwives, and Other Women's Healthcare Providers

Your office has been a source of comfort and advice throughout the pregnancy. This intimate relationship makes it likely that a woman experiencing distress will come to you for help. However, many women will not be forthcoming with negative feelings or concerns unless specifically asked. Women with a history of neonatal loss need monitoring and extra support. Have referrals to local professionals trained in perinatal mood disorders and information in the Resources section available. Please follow up on a regular basis.

A woman taking psychotropic medication who is pregnant or planning a pregnancy should be encouraged to consult a perinatal psychiatrist to determine whether to continue or change her medication. Women on medication for a bipolar disorder or psychosis should definitely be referred to a psychiatrist to develop a medication plan. These women need careful monitoring throughout pregnancy and postpartum.

We recommend you use a standardized postpartum screening tool. Women should be assessed throughout the first year. If your last visit to her is before one year postpartum, make sure she has referral information in case she needs it later.

Women already on medication, or those who you assess need a medical evaluation, should be referred to a psychiatrist specializing in perinatal mood and anxiety disorders.

Psychiatrists

Since you are the professionals who work most closely with psychotropic medications, many perinatal women will be referred to you for assessment and treatment of mood disorders. You play an integral role in this treatment team.

Research findings and recommendations about medications in pregnancy and lactation are constantly changing. There have been some important findings recently in the area of managing medication for perinatal mood and anxiety disorders, which are discussed later in this text. If you are only providing medication management, make sure you give your patients the name of a psychotherapist trained in PMADs. You can find skilled psychotherapists in the Resources section in the back of the book. It is essential to have a list of local resources and referrals.

Birth Doulas

Studies show that the use of a doula contributes to the reduction of postpartum depression. As a birth doula, you are in a unique position to screen prenatally for risk and to watch for early warning signs of emotional problems. If, for instance, when administering the Prepregnancy and Pregnancy Risk Assessment, you discover the woman has suffered a previous traumatic delivery or childhood sexual abuse, she may experience flashbacks during the upcoming birth. Have referrals to local professionals trained in perinatal mood disorders and information in the Resources section available.

A woman taking psychotropic medication who is pregnant or planning a pregnancy should be encouraged to consult a psychiatrist (specializing in PMADs) in order to determine whether to continue her medication. Recommendations will differ based on each woman's history. Women on medication for a bipolar disorder or psychosis should definitely be referred to a psychiatrist to develop a medication plan. These women need careful monitoring throughout pregnancy and postpartum.

If you are interviewed before employment, you can ask her if she has any particular concerns about birthing or postpartum. She then may share some information, which could give you clues about her mental health. Let the woman know that one of your strengths is sensitivity to the various emotions that can occur during birth and postpartum.

Use the Pre-pregnancy and Pregnancy Risk Assessment on *all* women who employ your services. If you continue to see these women postpartum, use the Postpartum Risk Assessment. Keep in mind that this information can be gathered quite informally, simply through chatting. Be familiar with the questions and the pertinent information you need in order to screen.

Postpartum Doulas and Visiting Nurses

You have the opportunity to observe the home and social environments of the mother, which can give crucial information about her well-being and that of the family unit. For instance, if you notice a lack of partner support or signs of marital conflict, she is at greater risk for a PMAD. If her house is unusually neat and clean, you will want to find out who is doing the housework. If she is, for example, obsessively cleaning or awake in the middle of the night vacuuming, this is not normal.

Help to create a healing and supportive environment, such as opening curtains to give more light, checking to see if she has healthful food, and eliminating unnecessary noise to make her home calmer and more soothing.

If you are just meeting women postpartum, you have not had the opportunity to screen them prenatally. We recommend you use a standardized postpartum screening tool such as the EPDS or the PDSS. Women should be assessed throughout the first year. If your last visit to her is before one year postpartum, make sure she has referral information in case she needs it later.

Women already on medication, or those who you assess need a medical evaluation, should be referred to a psychiatrist specializing in perinatal mood and anxiety disorders. Have referrals to local professionals trained in perinatal mood and anxiety disorders and information in the Resources section available.

Lactation Consultants

The role of a lactation consultant may superficially appear to be one-dimensional and relate only to the mechanics of breastfeeding. However, as we know, you are also providing tremendous emotional support. You may be the first professional to see the mother and baby during the initial postpartum weeks.

Your intimate relationship with the mother at this vulnerable time allows you to observe and listen for potential emotional problems. Postpartum moms listen carefully to what you advise and are quite trusting of you. It is so important that you help each woman decide what is right for her.

If her physical or emotional health is declining, it is obviously not good for the baby. You have a great deal of influence as to whether new mothers give themselves permission to take care of themselves (for instance, six hours of uninterrupted sleep at night, at least a few nights per week). A support person will need to feed the baby during this half of the night.

Breastfeeding difficulties may be associated with sexual abuse, childbirth trauma, OCD, depression, and anxiety. Women who are suffering with depression and anxiety give up breastfeeding more quickly. When their mental health improves, it often lengthens the duration of their breastfeeding. Sudden weaning can precipitate a mood or anxiety disorder, especially when a woman is predisposed. If she is already suffering, abrupt weaning can greatly exacerbate her symptoms. Especially if a woman is depressed and not feeling good about herself, there can be a great amount of guilt if at any point she cannot or should not continue breastfeeding. What you say or do not say at that time can make a big difference regarding how she feels about herself as a mother.

Many professionals are unaware of the current research regarding psychotropic medications in breast milk. It is important that you are informed so you can advocate for women who want to continue taking medication. Have referrals to local professionals trained in perinatal mood and anxiety disorders and information in the Resources section available, including a psychiatrist who has experience prescribing medication during lactation. We recommend you use a standardized postpartum screening tool. Women should be assessed throughout the first year. If your last visit with her is within one year postpartum, make sure she has referral information in case she needs it later.

Women already on medication, or those who you assess need a medical evaluation, should be referred to a psychiatrist specializing in perinatal mood and anxiety disorders.

Childbirth Educators

So often we hear the lament, "Why didn't anyone warn us in our birthing classes about mood and anxiety problems during and after pregnancy?" Even though your primary focus is on labor and delivery, you have a responsibility and opportunity to educate couples about perinatal mental illness. This might be a difficult topic to discuss since no woman wants to think it could happen to her.

If you know a professional who is an expert in this field, you can invite her or him to speak to your class. If not, bring the subject up in a matter-of-fact manner, the same way you would any other common pregnancy or postpartum experience.

The rate of depression in pregnancy is about 15 to 23 percent. Therefore, we can assume some of the women in your classes are already suffering and are at risk for a postpartum mood or anxiety disorder. Your participants will not bring up this topic, so you need to. There is no danger in giving information, and there is great danger in omitting it. Her partner might soak up this information even if the mother-to-be does not. It is often the spouse who later recognizes the symptoms and encourages his wife to seek help.

Hand out some information from the Resources section and the name and number of a professional trained in perinatal mood disorders. If you follow up with participants, ask about their feelings regarding the challenges as well as the joys of parenthood. Be sure to call participants who did not attend the reunion. They may not be doing well and could be trying to avoid an uncomfortable situation. The PSI DVD (listed in the "Resource" section) will be a helpful tool.

New Parent Group Leaders

If there are ten women in your group, remember that, statistically, one or two of them will have a PMAD. Rarely will this woman be brave enough to disclose her feelings, since she will most likely be experiencing guilt and shame. She will be aching for someone to open the door to this discussion and give her permission to express how she is really feeling. If partners are present, ask them how they themselves are doing. Dads/partners may have preexisting mood or anxiety disorders. The stress of a pregnancy can also worsen symptoms in them. No matter what, dads and partners need and deserve support too.

Encourage discussion about the normal feelings accompanying adjustment to parenting and the relationship to oneself, partner, baby, friends, and family. You can easily work in some facts about moods and behaviors that fall outside the realm of normal adjustment.

For each new group, make sure this topic gets explored in a non-judgmental manner. If you prefer, you can invite a professional with expertise in this area to lead a discussion. In any case, use the information in the Resources section and the names and numbers of local professionals trained in the area of postpartum disorders.

Adjunct Professionals

There are many other wonderful professionals who touch the lives of pregnant and postpartum women. For example, physical therapists and instructors in prenatal and postpartum exercise should mention the possibility of mood and anxiety disorders, since you are encountering suffering women all the time. Above all, making the information in the Resources section available will support the pregnant and postpartum women with whom you work.

Seven
Treatment

Why Is Treatment Necessary?

Science evolves and changes our beliefs and views. People used to believe the world was flat and that babies should sleep on their stomachs. Now we know the world is actually round, and putting babies to sleep on their backs reduces the risk of sudden infant death syndrome (SIDS). Research about perinatal mood and anxiety disorders has also taught us new things. In the past, people thought these illnesses didn't exist, or if they did, women didn't need treatment and should suffer through them, and that they would eventually recover on their own. We now know how incorrect that thinking was. Untreated illness in pregnancy will most likely lead to postpartum illness. At seven months postpartum, depression continues in up to 25 to 50 percent of women who are not treated. Untreated mood and anxiety disorders may go away after a time, but increase the likelihood of another episode or episodes later in life. Most people, if diagnosed with diabetes or cancer, would immediately seek treatment. Perinatal illnesses are not different— they require treatment and care. The brain is at least as important as any other part of the body.

Untreated mood and anxiety illnesses in pregnancy are associated with:

- Self-medication with potentially unsafe over-the-counter remedies, tobacco, alcohol, or drugs
- Poor nutrition and lack of self-care
- Appetite changes and abnormal weight gain or loss
- Poor fetal growth and low birth weight
- Premature birth
- Babies who cry more and are more difficult to soothe and calm

- Behavioral problems in preschoolers
- Developmental delays in toddlers
- Antisocial, aggressive, and violent behavior in teens

Moms who have untreated postpartum illness may:

- Have babies whose brain waves show depression
- Have difficulty with bonding and attachment
- Have babies who cry more
- Have children with poor language and cognitive (thinking) development and poor school readiness
- Be less likely to use car seats and are more likely to use harsh discipline
- Be less likely to start feeding with breast milk and less likely to continue
- Have children who are 50 percent more likely to suffer anxiety or depression when they become teens

It's also been shown that treating depression or anxiety in parents is not always enough to repair the alterations in the mother-infant or mother-child attachment and relationship. Special attention needs to be given to these relationships in the healing process. Activities that involve physical touch, such as infant massage, have been shown to be helpful. Professionals who work in this field include developmental psychologists and infant mental health specialists.

Untreated illness affects the whole family. You need and deserve to be well!

Research

Research doesn't always tell the whole story. There are lots of challenges understanding research. Here are some questions to ask:

Where is it reported?

Dr. Google is often not a reliable source. Forums and most blogs (we list a good one in the Resources section) are not scientific. Usually they contain individuals' personal stories. Even large well-respected news sources blur scientific conclusions to create attention-getting headlines.

How many people were studied?

The smaller the study population, the less meaningful the result. The most valuable studies have thousands of participants, or at least other research that repeats the results of the smaller study.

What was measured or studied? How was it measured?

For example, there are many studies of the effects of medication on the fetus. Some studies base results on prescriptions written, and then look at the infants. The problem? Just having a prescription, even if filled, does not always mean the woman actually took the medication. And even if she took the medication, she may not have taken the dose prescribed or necessary to treat her depression or anxiety.

Many studies that looked at the impact of medications on a fetus have not taken into account other critical factors that can impact outcomes, like cigarettes, drugs, alcohol, poor nutrition, or the effects of depression or anxiety if the woman was on an inadequate dose of medication. Genetic risk is also important to consider, for instance, when looking at autism.

Our goal is to translate and summarize the best studies to help you make the best decisions for you and your family.

Prevention

Prevention of a perinatal mood and anxiety disorder is, of course, the ultimate goal. Research is beginning to evaluate preventive methods. What follows is some of the best information currently available.

In a Canadian study, women at high risk for postpartum depression were offered an extended postpartum hospital stay (up to five days) in a private room. Their babies slept in the nursery at night so the moms could sleep without interruption. The moms also met once with a member of the Canadian Women's Health Concerns Clinic during their stay. This study highlighted the importance of uninterrupted sleep and support, as these women were less likely to suffer from postpartum depression, and for those who did get depressed, the depression was milder.

There are also studies showing that psychotherapy can be used effectively for prevention. Groups utilizing interpersonal psychotherapy, cognitive behavioral therapy, and psychoeducation during pregnancy reduce the occurrence of postpartum depression and anxiety.

What about medication? A study found that women at high risk who started sertraline (Zoloft) within fifteen hours after delivery significantly reduced their incidence of postpartum depression.

All new mothers need a wellness plan, because all moms need nurturing. This is not a luxury—it is a necessity! If a woman is at high risk, she should meet with a knowledgeable psychotherapist before pregnancy to create a prenatal and postpartum wellness plan. This plan may include follow-up appointments with other professionals such as a psychiatrist or nutritionist, sleep arrangements (to ensure blocks of uninterrupted sleep), food and eating (who will shop and cook), and getting breaks away from the baby during the week. If an illness occurs, a wellness plan will be in place that will support and speed recovery.

Information and education are critical components of treatment. Sometimes this is all a woman needs in order to recover. She needs to know her illness has a name and is treatable.

Treatment Guidelines

Pregnant and postpartum women need to be as symptom-free as possible. Pre-conception it may be reasonable to find or change to a medication that is low risk in pregnancy and of low concentration in breast milk. If a woman discovers she is pregnant and is doing well on a medication, the fetus has been exposed. The risk of illness due to changing medications is high. For every woman and caregiver, the risks of medication must always be weighed against the long-lasting risks of illness—on the mother, fetus, infant, and family. Always rule out bipolar disorder before giving antidepressants.

The goal of treatment, no matter what kind of treatment is chosen, is that the woman feels like herself again as quickly as possible.

Psychotherapy

Psychotherapy is talk therapy. A perinatal mental healthcare provider is someone who has had specific training in issues related to pregnancy and postpartum mood and anxiety disorders. Training in depression and anxiety in the general population is not enough and does not in itself make the provider qualified to treat the unique set of treatment issues in perinatal mood and anxiety disorders. Psychoeducation is an important part of perinatal therapy. Psychoeducation is offering information and explaining issues related to perinatal illness and treatment. A psychotherapist should be familiar with local resources as well as those on the web and in print. Psychotherapy can be done with the individual woman, with the couple, with family members, or in a group setting.

Pregnancy and postpartum treatment involves crisis management. The treatments found to be most effective specifically for perinatal mood and anxiety disorders are short-term or brief psychotherapies focused on symptom reduction and an improvement in functioning. This is not the time for long-term psychodynamic or psychoanalytic therapy. Two types or models of psychotherapy have been studied and have been shown to be effective for prevention and treatment of perinatal mood and anxiety disorders. These models are called Interpersonal Psychotherapy (IPT) and Cognitive-Behavioral Therapy (CBT). In both models the therapist plays an active role facilitating and directing discussion and teaching problem-solving skills. Both have been shown to be effective for the prevention and treatment of perinatal mood and anxiety disorders. Psychotherapy has been shown to have a long-lasting positive impact.

The Interpersonal Psychotherapy (IPT) model works to help clients address role changes, transitions and conflicts, and loss and grief, and build interpersonal skills as well as support resources.

Cognitive-Behavioral Therapy works by helping monitor and change thinking and behavior through education and skill building. CBT helps clients develop new ways to think and evaluate life experiences, and teaches practical tools that can be used immediately. Both models work on client strengths. When a woman is unable to process or apply psychotherapeutic strategies, medication is often indicated.

Social Support

Social support provides nonjudgmental empathetic emotional support, feedback, active listening, and information. Social support creates an environment where women can see that they are not alone or to blame. Social support often utilizes specially trained women who themselves have recovered from a perinatal mood or anxiety disorder. Social support can include emotional support as well as practical physical support. Support networks include support groups, telephone support, home visitors, email and online groups, faith communities, and family and friends.

Numerous studies have shown that a variety of social support models are effective in helping women recover. Contact Postpartum Support International (see the Resources section) to find social support.

Complementary and Alternative Therapies

Studies are currently being conducted regarding treatment in pregnancy and postpartum that do not involve prescription medication. For instance, the therapeutic effect of massage is beginning to emerge. Morning bright light therapy (natural sunlight or special light boxes) is already being used either as an alternative or in addition to medication. Exciting evidence about the effectiveness of the omega-3 essential fatty acids DHA (docosahexaenoic acid) and EPA (eicosapentaenoic acid) in both the prevention and treatment of prenatal and postpartum depression and anxiety is also apparent. The American Psychiatric Association recommends that patients with a mood disorder take 1 gm EPA plus DHA daily. These omega-3s are from fish oil, not the plant sources, which are different. At this point omega-3s are recommended to enhance, but not replace, standard treatment. Read the labels carefully to make sure you are getting both EPA and DHA. Be sure to talk with your healthcare provider before taking supplements of any kind. If you take omega-3s while nursing, the baby's neurological development may also be enhanced (these "lipophilic acids" have now been added to many baby formulas).

About 5 percent of pregnant women report using marijuana (cannabis). Cannabis is detectable in the placenta, amniotic fluid and the fetus. In a large study, maternal cannabis used during pregnancy was found to be associated with poor fetal growth in mid and late pregnancy, with effects on low birth weight being most noticeable if use continued throughout pregnancy. Even with legal medical marijuana, no "safe" dose has been established for perinatal use. There are increasing concerns about long-term neurodevelopmental, behavioral, and possibly even metabolic consequences of prenatal cannabis exposure.

Marijuana is also found in breast milk and may even be higher than that found in the mother's blood. Exposure through breast milk may affect brain development in children under 1 year of age. If you are using marijuana on a regular basis, we encourage you to speak with your healthcare provider. There are other well-researched ways to treat nausea, depression and anxiety.

Another new nonmedication treatment for depression is repetitive transcranial magnetic stimulation (TMS). TMS uses noninvasive brain stimulation and is showing great promise in the treatment of major depression. TMS is approved by the FDA for the treatment of major depressive disorder in adults, and a few small studies have been done on depressed pregnant women. Depression was reduced significantly within three weeks, and no ill effects were seen on the mom or baby. Certainly, more studies on safety need to be done, and TMS equipment is not yet widely available. TMS may be an effective therapy for women who choose not to go on medication. Be on the lookout for more information on this promising treatment.

A study at Stanford University found that acupuncture might be a helpful treatment for depression in pregnancy. Some insurance companies will pay for alternative treatment.

We advocate using the therapy or combination of therapies (including medication) that is the most effective for each individual. In other words, use whatever is known to be safe and works.

Women seeking treatment often try to reduce symptoms on their own before seeking the advice of a professional. This self-treatment may include potentially risky substances, such as alcohol or untested herbal or drug remedies. Twenty percent of pregnant women smoke, 19 percent use alcohol, and 6 percent use illegal drugs as a way to alter moods.

Herbs can be wonderful, but they can also be dangerous. Poisonous mushrooms are "natural," and digitalis, the heart medicine, is from a plant ("natural"). Little research has been done on the safety or effectiveness of herbs during pregnancy or nursing.

Very few studies have been done evaluating the safety of St. John's wort during pregnancy or in breast milk. There is no research that shows that St. John's wort is an effective treatment for anxiety or obsessive-compulsive disorder. St. John's wort interacts with a number of medications, including medications for heart disease, depression, seizures, certain cancers, and birth control pills. This means St. John's wort makes the birth control pill less effective. Herbal remedies are often produced with little or no regulation or safety monitoring. You cannot tell the quality or quantity of the active ingredient you're receiving in each dose. Because there is no governmental regulation on herbal preparations, studies have found that the measured amounts of the active ingredients varied considerably from those claimed on the labels, from 0 percent to 109 percent for capsules and from 31 percent to 80 percent for tablets.

This makes it impossible to know what and how much of the herb you're actually taking. Having a correct diagnosis is essential before starting any kind of treatment. For instance, like an antidepressant, SAMe, St. John's wort, and bright light therapy can all trigger hypomania or mania in women with bipolar illness.

There have been a number of articles in the media recently reporting stories of women who claim that eating their placenta after a birth prevents postpartum blues and possibly protects against postpartum depression and anxiety. Placenta eating has been part of cultural rituals around the world. And, indeed, some animal species do eat the placenta after birth, but we don't know the reason or value. Unfortunately, no one has measured the emotional health of women or animals that do eat their placenta. As of mid-2015, there are still no studies that have been reported on the effectiveness or benefits of placenta ingestion and mood in humans. The information shown as "research" by advocates of placental encapsulation does not contain one study evaluating human ingestion and mood, energy or hormone levels. Remember that 30 percent of people will feel better when given a placebo or "sugar pill."

On the other hand, quite a bit of research has been conducted regarding the use and effectiveness of certain prescription medications during pregnancy and lactation that effectively combat and treat perinatal mood and anxiety disorders. These prescription medications are monitored by the Food and Drug Administration (FDA) to make sure there are no contaminants, and that the dose is indeed the stated dose.

For many years the FDA used a confusing and misleading rating scale for safety labeling of medication during pregnancy. The old categories used a rating system labeling medications A, B, C, D, or X. For example, medications with less research were often labeled safer, while medications that often had more research were sometimes labeled less safe, regardless of the outcome of the studies. As of June 2015, that old system will be discarded and replaced by a more informative safety labeling of medications used during pregnancy and in breast milk.

The most immediate goal of treatment is to alleviate suffering as quickly as possible. While it is general practice to start medication at a low dosage, it should be increased as rapidly as possible to whatever the right dosage is for that woman. Undertreating can lead to chronic problems and suffering, and increases the risk of relapse.

What follows here are guidelines only. All treatment must be individualized. For medication management we recommend you see a psychiatrist with expertise in treating perinatal illnesses. No matter what treatments you choose, someone with expertise should monitor you. Be persistent! If one practitioner or provider, or one medication or treatment method doesn't work or feel like a good fit, try another. The goal is to feel like you again. Feeling "OK" or "better" is not good enough.

Pregnancy and Medication

Current thinking regarding the use of medications in pregnancy has evolved over the past few years. Researchers who have spent years investigating the potential effects of medication on the fetus have shifted their focus to the harmful effects on the fetus when maternal mental illness goes untreated. These experts agree that maternal depression and anxiety must be evaluated and treated to maximize a positive outcome for the baby and the mother. When evaluating risks of medication in pregnancy, it is critical to remember that all normal pregnancies have a 3 to 5 percent chance of a birth defect. Pregnancy causes changes in metabolism and blood volume; therefore, higher doses of medications may be required to achieve an adequate reduction in symptoms. One study found that in order to remain symptom-free, two-thirds of women required an increase in dosage at six and a half months into the pregnancy.

In 2012, the *American Journal of Ob/Gyn* stated that when a psychiatric condition requires medication, the benefits of medication far outweigh potential minimal risks of medication. In the same year, the *American Journal of Psychiatry* published an article stating that not prescribing antidepressants to a woman who is depressed or likely to become ill again during pregnancy may cause more risks to the mom and fetus than the risks of exposure to medication.

Following is a summary of commonly used prescription medications for perinatal mood and anxiety disorders.

Antianxiety Medications

While the SSRIs are often used to treat anxiety, panic and OCD, it can sometimes take several weeks before a reduction in symptoms is noticed. Another group of medications, the benzodiazepines, are used for immediate relief of anxiety. Taken over time, on a regular basis, these medications are addictive. We often find that women are so worried about becoming addicted, they don't take enough to adequately control their symptoms. These medications can be used for occasional episodes of anxiety. Sometimes they are used with SSRIs to keep anxiety under control, usually on a short-term basis. Alprzolam (Xanax) and lorazepam (Ativan) are shorter acting (out of your system more quickly), while diazepam (Valium) and clonazepam (Klonopin) are longer acting.

The literature regarding antianxiety medications (*benzodiazepines*) during pregnancy is limited. For many years there was a concern that benzodiazepine exposure increased the risk of birth defects, particularly cleft lip and palate. There is now some evidence that maternal anxiety may itself contribute to cleft lip and palate birth defects. New research suggests the risk of birth defects in the first trimester is very low, and these medications can be used without concerns about birth defects in the second and third trimesters. Babies born to women taking high doses at the end of pregnancy may experience some temporary problems. However, women with anxiety or panic disorder should be treated. The lowest effective dose for the shortest period of time is recommended.

Antidepressants

Since we receive so many antidepressant questions from our pregnant clients (and those on medications who are considering another pregnancy), we have addressed some of the biggest concerns here. Brand names may vary by country, so we are including both brand and generic names of medications.

Do antidepressants cause miscarriage?

In a 2013 review and analysis of over 735 studies, it was found the risk of miscarriage was the same in women with depression as women who took antidepressants for depression. Studies of antidepressants have revealed that neither selective serotonin reuptake inhibitors (SSRIs) nor tricyclics (TCAs) pose any increased risk.

Can antidepressants cause prematurity?

A large review of studies in 2013 found no difference in prematurity rates in women on antidepressants compared to depressed women not on medication.

Does antidepressant use in pregnancy cause birth defects?

In all births there is a 1 to 3 percent chance of birth defects. Large studies in 2013 looked at many antidepressant medications including buproprion (Wellbutrin), citalopram (Celexa), fluoxetine (Prozac), paroxetine (Paxil), escitalopram (Lexapro) mirtazapine (Remeron), sertraline (Zoloft), venlafaxine (Effexor), fluvoxamine (Luvox), and nefazadone (Serzone) found that *antidepressant use even in the first trimester* was not associated with an increased risk of birth defects. There is a growing body of research on the safety of duloxetine (Cymbalta) and venlifaxine (Effexor). These new studies support previous findings made by The American Psychiatric Association and the American College of OB/GYNs who published a joint report in 2009. They summarized that there is no consistent evidence showing risk of stillbirths or birth defects with the use of SSRIs and other antidepressants. Also in 2009, the Mayo Clinic published a review of over 25,000 deliveries. Over 800 of those women were on antidepressant medication. All the women in the study had birth-defect rates below 1 percent, yet the women on medication for depression had lower rates of birth defects than the women not on medication. None of the babies exposed to medication had pulmonary hypertension (see next section), while 16 of the babies not exposed to medication did. The study concluded that the data was very reassuring about using SSRIs during pregnancy. Also, in 2009, the Motherisk Program (which studies medications that cause birth defects) found that antidepressant use even in the first trimester is not associated with an increased risk for major malformations above the level seen in all mothers.

What about Persistent Pulmonary Hypertension of the Newborn and antidepressants?

Persistent Pulmonary Hypertension of the Newborn (PPHN) occurs in about 0.1 percent of newborns. It is rare, but serious. Studies from 2009 and 2010 did not show an increase in PPHN in babies exposed to SSRIs during pregnancy. It was noted in 2012 that many of the known risk factors for PPHN such as obesity, smoking, shorter pregnancies, and cesarean birth are more commonly seen in depressed women.

Do antidepressants cause poor neonatal adaptation or withdrawal?

This refers to symptoms (often breathing problems) that are sometimes seen in newborns whose moms are on medication during the last trimester of pregnancy. It is unclear if this is caused by too much serotonin (a brain chemical) in the baby, or a withdrawal from the medication. Reported rates vary from 10 to 30 percent, and seem more common in women who take paroxetine (Paxil). The symptoms begin in the first few days of life, and usually are gone within 3–5 days. A joint report of The American Psychiatric Association and the American College of OB/GYNs notes that discontinuing medication to avoid symptoms in the newborn may lead to relapse in the mother. *This is a mild syndrome that most often does not require treatment. It goes away by itself. Stopping medication in the last trimester puts a mother at a greater risk of depression at the end of pregnancy and during her postpartum course.*

Do antidepressants cause autism?

One study in 2011 was reported wildly in the media, linking SSRI use with Autism Spectrum Disorder. This study looked at a very small group and looked at women who were written one prescription for an SSRI the year before the pregnancy. The research did not take into account a family or personal history of autism or mental illness, both major risk factors for autism. The authors conclude their report by saying that prenatal SSRI exposure is not a major risk for autism. In a much bigger study conducted in Denmark in 2013, no association was found between prenatal exposure to antidepressant medication and autism in the children.

Has anyone found problems in older children exposed to antidepressant medication during pregnancy?

In a study of children tested at ages 3 to 7, IQ and development tests were all normal. This included first-trimester exposure. It was found that severity of maternal depression during pregnancy predicted children's behavior problems. The IQ of the mom and the sex of the child predicted the child's IQ. The use of antidepressants and the dose or length of time taken, were not predictors of cognitive or behavioral problems. Another study looking at children 4 to 5 years of age found that prenatal antidepressant use was not associated with behavioral or emotional problems in early childhood.

If you are already on an antidepressant, remember that discontinuing your medication before delivery, a time that is high risk for depression and anxiety, can put you at significant risk for illness. Speak to someone who knows the research before you make any changes in your medication. In addition, the top researchers maintain that there is no reason to change from one antidepressant to another. Go with what works and gets the quickest results.

Antipsychotics

These drugs are also called *major tranquilizers.* Older high-potency antipsychotics such as haloperidol (Haldol) have been recommended in the past over low-potency or atypical agents throughout pregnancy. Now there is a little more information about the newer atypical antipsychotics. One long-term study found children age 4 who were exposed during pregnancy had normal IQs. No increased risk of birth defects or complications have been seen in studies of the newer atypical antipsychotic medications olanzapine (Zyprexa), risperidone (Risperdal), or quetiapine (Seroquel). These newer drugs seem to have fewer side effects, although they may increase weight gain.

If you are considering taking one of these medications during pregnancy, please sign up with the National Pregnancy Registry for Atypical Antipsychotics. This will add to the information about the care of women treated with this class of agents who are either attempting to conceive or pregnant: womensmental-health.org/clinical-and-research-programs/pregnancyregistry/.

Electroconvulsive Therapy (ECT)

ECT is considered an acceptable treatment for severe depression or psychosis in pregnancy. It may also be useful in treating bipolar disorder during pregnancy. ECT is not used for prenatal anxiety, panic, or obsessive-compulsive disorder (OCD).

Mood Stabilizers

Women with bipolar disorder should consider continuing on medication throughout pregnancy, because the danger of relapse is so high. Twenty-four percent of women with a history of chronic bipolar disorder became ill during pregnancy even while on medication, so stopping medication is obviously quite risky. A study of bipolar women who discontinued mood stabilizers when they became pregnant was reported at an American Psychiatric Association meeting. Within three months, half of the women relapsed, and by six months, about 70 percent had relapsed. Restarting lithium after stopping it in the first trimester does not protect well against relapse.

Medications used for seizure disorders are often used as mood stabilizers in women with bipolar disorder. Valproate (Depakote) can cause serious birth defects, and its use is not widely recommended for women of childbearing age. Lamotrigine (Lamictal), also an antiseizure medication, is now considered the antiepileptic drug of choice for pregnant women.

Lithium is an antimania medication used to treat bipolar disorders. Recent research shows that the risk of Ebstein's anomaly (a heart defect in fetuses) with lithium use in the first trimester is only about one to two per thousand. A fetal cardiac ultrasound between weeks 18 and 20 is recommended for those with first-trimester exposure. No significant neurobehavioral or developmental problems have been reported in children who were exposed to lithium during pregnancy. Other mood stabilizers, such as carbamazepine (Tegretol) and valproic acid (Depakote), increase the rate of neural tube defects and other birth defects. Children examined at 3 years of age were found to have decreased IQ when exposed to Tegretol during pregnancy. Because of this, an increased dose of folic acid is often used in addition to Tegretol or Depakote if either of these medications must be continued.

Ideally, women on these medications should consult with a psychiatrist familiar with the latest research before getting pregnant to plan how to best manage their illness during the course of a pregnancy.

Sleep Aids

Depression and anxiety can cause problems falling or staying asleep. Sleep is an essential part of the treatment plan. Sometimes medication may be necessary. There are several over-the-counter medications that are considered fine to use while pregnant. These are doxylamine (Unisom) and diphendramamine (Benadryl).

Trazadone (Deseryl) and amitriptyline (Elavil) are antidepressants that have a sedative effect. Zolpidem (Ambien) has a faster rate of onset and is considered acceptable in pregnancy. When anxiety is contributing to sleep difficulty and other methods are not effective, antianxiety medications such as Ativan or Xanax can be quite helpful.

Postpartum

The birth of a baby may bring about the need to change the medication treatment plan. While a growing fetus is exposed to higher doses of maternal medication, a few medications can be problematic for infants receiving breast milk. Some women may choose to restart or begin medication after the birth. Most medications are found in low levels in breast milk, and are considered very low risk to the infant.

Thyroid

At least 10 percent of postpartum women will develop postpartum thyroiditis. In the early stages of thyroiditis, women may experience anxiety or depression. Sometimes this condition is temporary and will go away without treatment in about six months. But for others it can lead to chronic thyroiditis and hypothyroidism (Hashimoto's thyroiditis).

Since thyroid disorders can cause depression and anxiety, ask your provider to check your blood. The suggested time for testing is between two and three months postpartum. The following tests are recommended for all women with postpartum mood complaints: free T4, TSH, anti-TPO, and antithyroglobulin. It is important to check for the antithyroid antibodies (anti-TPO and antithyroglobulin) since there have been many cases where the T4 and TSH levels were within normal ranges but the antithyroid antibody levels were elevated. If thyroid labs are abnormal, we recommend that women be evaluated by an endocrinologist.

Hormone Therapy

Hormone therapy for postpartum depression is still being evaluated for effectiveness. Research with estrogen holds promise for treatment of postpartum depression and postpartum psychosis. Taking estrogen, like any medicine, has certain risks and needs to be evaluated on a case-by-case basis. It appears that it is not a low level of hormones that seems to cause mood problems for most postpartum women. Rather, it's the shifting of hormone levels that women are sensitive to.

Women sensitive to hormonal shifts, including those with postpartum depression and anxiety who choose oral contraceptives (birth control pills), need to be monitored closely for mood changes. Women may experience fewer mood problems on a monophasic birth control pill as compared to a triphasic birth control pill. The monophasic pill delivers the same ratio of estrogen and progesterone, unlike the triphasic, in which the ratio changes weekly.

Women with a history of increased moodiness on oral contraceptives should consider alternate methods of contraception. Synthetic progesterone (progestin) including the "minipill" has been associated with a worsening of symptoms. Medroxyprogesterone acetate (Depo-Provera), a long-acting progesterone injection, is not a good option since it cannot be discontinued should it aggravate mood problems. There have also been reports of mood problems after insertion of the progesterone releasing IUD. These mood problems quickly resolve once the IUD is removed. Hormone therapy is not recommended, at this time, as sole treatment for postpartum psychiatric disorders. Currently, research has started looking at the use of an estrogen patch as a form of treatment for postpartum depression.

Medications

If you or a blood relative has had a positive experience with any particular medication, that would be the first choice. Few studies have been done on the effectiveness any one particular medication over another in the treatment of postpartum depression/anxiety. One study found venlafaxine (Effexor) and another found sertraline (Zoloft) to be effective in the treatment of postpartum depression. Bupropion (Wellbutrin) for postpartum women with depression but without anxiety seems to be energizing and also reduces the likelihood of sexual side effects.

There is not one medication that, in general, is better than the others for treating postpartum depression and anxiety. The "best" one for each woman is the one that works for her. In our experience all the SSRIs work well. Each woman has her own individual chemistry, which will work better with certain medications than with others. It is recommended that a woman start SSRIs at a low dose with regular follow-up, increasing the dosage until an adequate therapeutic response is achieved. Treatment of anxiety, including obsessive-compulsive disorder, usually requires a higher dosage. She should report feeling 100 percent "back to herself." Just feeling better is not good enough. Undertreating can lead to chronic illness and increased risk of relapse.

Medications and Breast Milk

Giving a baby breast milk has great benefits for both the baby and mother. For some women, breast milk may feel like the only positive thing they have to offer the baby. Most medications for depression and anxiety are found in very low amounts in breast milk and in the babies. There are, however, a few medications that are not recommended or must be used with caution.

Antianxiety Medications

Low doses of short-acting medications such as alprazolam (Xanax) or lorazepam (Ativan) can be used on an occasional as-needed basis for anxiety, panic, and poor sleep. A study reported in the *Journal of Pediatrics* in 2012 concluded it was acceptable to take benzodiazepines (antianxiety medications) while feeding with breast milk. No adverse effects were seen in infants over two weeks of age.

Antidepressants

Of the most commonly used antidepressants, sertraline (Zoloft) and paroxetine (Paxil) were detected in the smallest amounts in the infant. Fluoxetine (Prozac), citalopram (Celexa), and escitalopram (Lexapro) were found in small amounts in the infant's blood, and no significant problems were noted in the infants. These babies were rechecked at a year and a half and found to have normal development and IQ. It is generally felt that it is safe to feed with breast milk while taking antidepressants. The first choice for every woman should be a medication that has worked for her in the past or one that has been used successfully with a blood relative.

The benefits of breast milk far outweigh any known risks of medications. Behaviorally and developmentally, these infants and children are normal.

Antipsychotics

Also called *major tranquilizers*, these medications are used to treat psychosis and also are used to treat women suffering from severe anxiety. They also enhance the effectiveness of SSRIs. High-potency antipsychotics, such as haloperidol (Haldol), are used for moms feeding with breast milk. The babies should be watched for sleepiness; however, there have been no reports of infant problems. The "second generation" or atypical antipsychotics olanzapine (Zyprexa), risperidone (Risperdal), or quetiapine (Seroquel) are seen in very small amounts in breast milk, and considered compatible.

Electroconvulsive Therapy (ECT)

ECT is considered an acceptable treatment for severe depression or psychosis postpartum, and does not affect breast milk. It may also be useful in treating bipolar disorder postpartum. ECT is not used for postpartum anxiety, panic, or OCD.

Mood Stabilizers

The safety of taking carbamazepine (Tegretol) or valproate (Depakote) while feeding with breast milk is undecided. Consult your healthcare practitioner for guidance. In the past, women were told they should not give the baby breast milk if they were taking lithium. Small studies have shown little risk to the infant. However, babies need to have blood tests to monitor lithium levels. Lamotrigine (Lamictal) is considered acceptable while feeding with breast milk.

Sleep Aids

Zolpidem (Ambien), temazepam (Restoril), trazadone (Deseryl), nortriptyline (Pamelor), and amitriptyline (Elavil) are frequently prescribed for moms feeding with breast milk.

Medical Protocols

The guidelines on the next pages suggest treatments based upon the woman's history. Treatments should be followed in sequence, with Treatment 1 tried first, followed by Treatment 2 if necessary.

Although the treatment protocols that follow refer only to depression and psychosis, they are also effective in the treatment of OCD, anxiety, and panic.

SSRIs are usually the first choice in the treatment of OCD, anxiety, and panic. It may be helpful to use low-dose antianxiety or antipsychotic medications on a short-term basis for anxiety and panic. Often high doses of SSRIs are needed, and for longer periods of time.

PREPREGNANCY		
History	**Treatment 1**	**Treatment 2**
One episode of major depression if on medication + asymptomatic for 6–12 months	Taper off medication + psychotherapy (monitor closely for relapse) + social support	Resume medication + continue psychotherapy + social support
Severe recurrent prior episodes	Continue medication + psychotherapy + social support	Psychotherapy + medication + social support
Mild major depression or severe major depression (first episode)	Psychotherapy + social support	Psychotherapy + medication + social support
Bipolar disorder	Continue or switch if on valproic acid (Depakote) or carbamazepine (Tegretol) to lithium or Lamotrigine (Lamictal) + have psychiatrist monitor closely + psychotherapy + social support	Switch to high potency antipsychotic if necessary + continue psychotherapy + social support when stable

PREGNANCY (including first trimester)		
History	**Treatment 1**	**Treatment 2**
One episode mild major depression, currently in remission	Try slowly tapering medication + psychotherapy + social support	Resume medication + psychotherapy + social support
One episode severe major depression, currently in remission	If stable consider slow tapering off or maintenance of medication + psychotherapy + social support	Medication + psychotherapy + social support if relapse
Mild major depression, first or recurrent	Psychotherapy + social support	Medication + psychotherapy + social support
Severe major depression, first episode	Medication + psychotherapy + social support	ECT + psychotherapy
Recurrence or relapse of depression if off medication if mild major depression	Psychotherapy + social support	Resume medication + psychotherapy + social support
Severe major depression, currently symptomatic	Resume medication + psychotherapy + social support	ECT + psychotherapy + social support
Psychosis in any trimester **Note:** Do not rely on psychosocial interventions alone; requires hospitalization.	Antipsychotic, add mood stabilizer or antidepressant if needed once stable; psychotherapy when stable Or ECT + psychotherapy	Hospitalization

POSTPARTUM		
Diagnosis	**Treatment 1**	**Treatment 2**
Mild major depression/anxiety	Psychotherapy + social support	Psychotherapy + medication + social support
Severe major depression/anxiety	Psychotherapy + medication + social support	Consider addition of atypical antipsychotic
Postpartum psychosis **Note:** Hospitalization required; do not rely on psychosocial interventions alone.	Antipsychotic + psychotherapy once stable	Consider ECT

PREVENTION OF POSTPARTUM DEPRESSION IN WOMEN WITH HISTORY OF DEPRESSION, ANXIETY, OTHER MOOD DISORDER, OR PRIOR POSTPARTUM ILLNESS		
History	Treatment 1	Treatment 2
First pregnancy	Meet with psychotherapist when risk identified (prepregnancy or pregnancy) + psychoeducation for woman and partner	Intervention (refer to pregnancy treatment protocol) if symptomatic
Prior postpartum depression/anxiety	Psychoeducation for woman and partner as early as possible + consider starting antidepressant (SSRI) 2-4 weeks before delivery or at delivery + psychotherapy	Intervention (refer to pregnancy treatment protocol) if symptomatic
Prior postpartum psychosis	Refer to psychiatrist, start antipsychotic upon delivery + psychotherapy	Intervention (refer to pregnancy treatment protocol) if symptomatic

Resources

Websites and Helplines

Childbirth and Postpartum Professional Association
CAPPA.net (United States)
Doula training and locating a doula.

CAPPAcanada.ca (Canada)
Training doulas and finding support.

Doulas of North America
dona.org
An international, nonprofit organization of doulas that strives to have every doula trained and educated to provide the highest quality and standards for birth and/or postpartum support to birthing women and their families.

infantrisk.org
Thomas Hale's website on medications in pregnancy and lactation from Texas Tech University Health Sciences Center.

The Marcé Society
marcesociety.com
The Marcé Society is an international organization dedicated to scientific research in the field. Annual conference.

Massachusetts General Hospital Center for Women's Mental Health
womensmentalhealth.org
A perinatal and reproductive psychiatry information center.

Motherisk
motherisk.org
1-877-439-2744
Provides expert information and guidance to women and their healthcare providers regarding medication exposure during pregnancy and postpartum. This website also has a section on morning sickness in pregnancy. Offers toll-free help-lines.

MotherToBaby

Mothertobaby.org

1-866-626-6847

Dedicated to providing evidence-based information to mothers, healthcare professionals, and the general public about medications and other exposures during pregnancy and while breastfeeding.

North American Society for Psychosocial OB/GYN

naspog.org

The North American Society for Psychosocial Obstetrics and Gynecology is a society of researchers, clinicians, educators, and scientists involved in women's mental health and healthcare. Outstanding conferences.

Pec Indman's Website

pecindman.com

Information about Dr. Indman and resources.

Postpartum Progress Blog

postpartumprogress.com

Award-winning blog on postpartum depression and other mental illnesses related to childbirth by survivor Katherine Stone. She covers news stories and resources.

Postpartum Support International (PSI)

postpartum.net

1-800-944-4PPD (944-4773)

Postpartum Support International is dedicated to helping women suffering from perinatal mood and anxiety disorders, including postpartum depression, the most common complication of childbirth. PSI works to educate family friends, and healthcare providers. The PSI motto is: You are not alone. You are not to blame. With help, you will be well. PSI offers telephone support and an international directory of members. The annual conference offers training for health professionals and consumers. PSI offers a standardized two-day curriculum as well as custom trainings. *Healthy Mom, Happy Family*, a thirteen-minute educational DVD in English and Spanish, are available at postpartum.net.

Shoshana Bennett's Website
DrShosh.com
Resources such as film *Dark Side of The Full Moon*
DarkSideoftheFullMoon.com and free app PPDGone!

Postpartum Dads/Partners
These sites offer support for dads, husbands and partners.

postpartumdads.org

postpartummen.com

Apps

Infant Risk Mobile App for Healthcare Providers
By Thomas Hale (author of *Medications in Mother's Milk*)
Texas Tech University Health Sciences Center

MommyMeds Pregnancy Safety Guide
By Texas Tech University Health Sciences Center

PPDGone!
Dr. Shoshana Bennett's free app with videos, audios, and articles related to prevention and treatment of perinatal mood and anxiety disorders

text4baby.org
Provides a free app offering 3 free text messages per week throughout your pregnancy and until your baby is one year old. These messages are about physical and emotional health during pregnancy and postpartum for the mom and infant.

Books

Beck, Cheryl, and Jeanne Driscoll. *Postpartum Mood and Anxiety Disorders: A Guide.* Sudbury, MA: Jones & Bartlett Publishers, 2005.

Beck, Cheryl, and Jeanne Driscoll. *Traumatic Childbirth.* New York, NY: Routledge, 2013.

Bennett, Shoshana. *Children of the Depressed: Healing the Childhood Wounds That Come from Growing Up with a Depressed Parent.* Oakland, CA: New Harbinger Publications, 2014.

Bennett, Shoshana. *Postpartum Depression for Dummies.* Indianapolis, IN: Wiley Publishing, Inc., 2007.

Bennett, Shoshana. *Pregnant on Prozac.* Guilford, CT: The Globe Pequot Press, 2009.

Chan, Paul D. *Why Is Mommy Sad? A Child's Guide to Parental Depression.* Laguna Hills, CA: Current Clinical Strategies Publishing, 2006.

Cohen, Lee, and Ruta Nonacs, eds. *Mood and Anxiety Disorders During Pregnancy and Postpartum.* Washington, DC: American Psychiatric Publishing, 2005.

Cox John, et al. *Perinatal Mental Health: The Edinburgh Postnatal Depression Scale (EPDS) Manual 2nd Ed.* London, England: The Royal College of Psychiatrists, 2014.

Dunnewold, Ann, and Diane Sanford. *Life Will Never Be the Same: A Real Moms Postpartum Survival Guide.* Dallas, TX: Real Moms Ink LLC, 2010.

Fran, Renee. *What Happened to Mommy?* R. D. Eastman Publishing, 1994. (Can be ordered on Amazon.com.)

Honikman, Jane. As the Founder of Postpartum Support International and an important figure in this field, her books can be found on JaneHonikman.com.

Honikman, Jane. *Community Support for New Families, A Guide to Organizing a Postpartum Parent Support Network in Your Community.* Santa Barbara, CA. *Community Support for New Families* is your guide to organizing a postpartum parent support network in your community.

Honikman, Jane. *I'm Listening: A Guide to Supporting Postpartum Families.* Santa Barbara, CA. *I'm Listening* teaches concerned, caring individuals how to help people struggling with postpartum depression (PPD) over the phone.

Karraa, Walker. *Transformed by Postpartum Depression: Women's Stories of Trauma and Growth.* Amarillo, TX: Praeclarus Press, 2014.

Kleiman, Karen. *The Postpartum Husband.* Philadelphia, PA: Xlibris, 2000.

Kleiman, Karen. *Therapy and the Postpartum Woman.* New York, NY: Routledge, 2009.

Kleiman, Karen. *What Am I Thinking? Having a Baby After Postpartum Depression.* Philadelphia, PA: Xlibris, 2005.

Kleiman, Karen, and Amy Wenzel. *Cognitive Behavioral Therapy for Perinatal Distress.* New York, NY: Routledge, 2014.

Kleiman, Karen, and Amy Wenzel. *Dropping the Baby and Other Scary Thoughts: Breaking the Cycle of Unwanted Thoughts in Motherhood.* New York, NY: Routledge, 2010.

Kleiman, Karen, and Amy Wenzel. *Tokens of Affection: Reclaiming Your Marriage After Postpartum Depression.* New York, NY: Routledge, 2014.

Kleiman, Karen, and Valerie Raskin. *This Isn't What I Expected* [2nd edition]: *Overcoming Postpartum Depression.* Boston, MA: Da Capo Lifelong Books, 2013.

Nicholson, et al. *Parenting Well When You're Depressed; A Complete Resource For Maintaining a Healthy Family.* Oakland, CA: New Harbinger Publications, Inc., 2001.

O'Reilly, Carla, et al. *The Smiling Mask: Truths about Postpartum Depression and Parenthood.* Regina, SK: To the Core Consulting, 2008.

Poulin, Sandra. *The Mother-to-Mother Postpartum Depression Support Book.* New York, NY: Berkley Trade, 2006.

Spinelli, Margaret G. *Infanticide: Psychosocial and Legal Perspectives on Mothers Who Kill.* Arlington, VA: American Psychiatric Publishing, 2002.

Twomey, Teresa. *Understanding Postpartum Psychosis; A Temporary Madness.* Westport, CT: Praeger Publishers, 2009.

Wiegartz, Pamela, and Kevin Gyoerkoe. *The Pregnancy & Postpartum Anxiety Workbook.* Oakland, CA: New Harbinger Publications, 2009.

Resources for Neonatal Loss

griefwatch.com

handonline.org

missfoundation.org

nationalshare.org

The following books are also recommended:

Blanford, Cathy. *Something Happened.* Western Springs, IL: Blanford, 2008. somethinghappenedbook.com. A book for children and parents who have experienced pregnancy loss.

Cohn, Janice. *Molly's Rosebush.* Park Ridge, IL: Albert Whitman & Company, 1994. For children 4–7.

Cirulli Lanham, Carol. *Pregnancy After a Loss: A Guide to Pregnancy After a Miscarriage, Stillbirth, or Infant Death.* New York, NY: Berkley Trade, 1999.

Davis, Deborah. *Empty Cradle, Broken Heart, Revised Edition: Surviving the Death of Your Baby.* Golden, CO: Fulcrum Publishing, 1996.

Lothrop, Hannah. *Help, Comfort, and Hope After Losing Your Baby in Pregnancy Or The First Year.* Cambridge, MA: Da Capo Press, 2004.

Nelson, Tim. *A Guide for Fathers: When A Baby Dies.* St. Paul, MN: Timothy Nelson. Revised 2007 edition.

Journal Articles

The articles listed in this section were written for medical professionals such as doctors and nurses. They are presented here for those readers who are comfortable with medical and scientific terminology.

Abramowitz, J. A. "Obsessive-Compulsive Symptoms in Pregnancy and the Puerperium: A Review of the Literature." *Anxiety Disorders* 2003; 17:461–478.

Altshuler, L., et al. "Pharmacologic Management of Psychiatric Illness During Pregnancy: Dilemmas and Guidelines." *American Journal of Psychiatry* 1996 May; 153:592–606.

Alwan S., et al. "National Birth Defects Prevention, Study. Use of Selective Serotonin-Reuptake Inhibitors in Pregnancy and the Risk of Birth Defects." *New England Journal of Medicine* 2007; 356:2684–2692.

American Academy of Pediatrics. "Use of Psychoactive Medication During Pregnancy and Possible Effects on the Fetus and Newborn." *Pediatrics* 2000 Apr; 105(4):880–887.

American College of OB/GYN Practice Bulletin. Use of Psychiatric Medications During Pregnancy and Lactation, 2008 April; No. 92.

Anderson, E., and I. Reti. "ECT in Pregnancy: A Review of the Literature from 1941–2007." *Psychosomatic Medicine* 2009; 71:235–242.

Andrade C. "The Safety of Duloxetine During Pregnancy and Lactation." *The Journal of Clinical Psychiatry* 2014 Dec; 75(12):e1423–7.

Appleby, L., et al. "A Controlled Study of Fluoxetine and Cognitive Behavioural Counseling in the Treatment of Postnatal Depression." *British Medical Journal* 1997; 314:932–936.

Beck, C. T. "Impact of Birth Trauma on Breastfeeding." *Nursing Research* 2008; 57(4):228–236.

Beck, C. T. "Maternal Depression and Child Behavior Problems: A Meta-Analysis." *Journal of Advanced Nursing* 1999; 29:623–629.

Beck, C. T., and Pec Indman. "The Many Faces of Postpartum Depression." *Journal of Obstetric, Gynecologic, & Neonatal Nursing* 2005; 34:569–576.

Beck, C. T., and R. Gable. "Postpartum Depression Screening Scale (PDSS)." Available through Western Psychological Services 1-800-648–8857.

Bennett, H. A. "Prevalence of Depression During Pregnancy. Systematic Review." *American College of OB/GYN* April 2004;103:698–709.

Bennett H. A., et al. "Prevalence of Depression During Pregnancy. Overview of Clinical Factors." *Clinical Drug Investigations* 2004; 24 (3): 157-179.

Bergink, V., et al. "Prevention of Postpartum Psychosis and Mania in Women at High Risk." *American Journal of Psychiatry* 2012; 169:609–15.

Berle, J. O., et al. "Neonatal Outcomes in Offspring of Women with Anxiety and Depression During Pregnancy." *Archives of Women's Mental Health* 2005; 8:181–189.

Birnbaum, C. S., et al. "Serum Concentrations of Antidepressants and Benzodiazepines in Nursing Infants: A Case Series." *Pediatrics* 1999; 104:11.

Bodnar, L., and Katherine Wisner. "Nutrition and Depression: Implications for Improving Mental Health Among Childbearing-Aged Women." *Biological Psychiatry* 2005; 58:679–685.

Borja-Hart, N. L., and Jehan Marino. "Role of Omega-3 Fatty Acids for Prevention or Treatment of Perinatal Depression." *Pharmacotherapy* 2010; 30(2):210–216.

Borri, C., et al. "Axis I Psychopathology and Functional Impairment at the Third Month of Pregnancy: Results from the Perinatal Depression-Research and Screening Unit (PND-ReScU) Study." *The Journal of Clinical Psychiatry* 2008; 69:1617–1624.

Boyd, R. C., et al. "Review of Screening Instruments for Postpartum Depression." *Archives of Women's Mental Health* 2005; 8(3):141–53.

Brandon, A. R., et al. "Nonpharmacologic Treatments for Depression Related to Reproductive Events." *Current Psychiatry Reports* October 2014, 16:526.

Byatt N., et al. "Antidepressant Use in Pregnancy: a Critical Review Focused on Risks and Controversies." *Acta Psychiatrica Scandinavica* 2013; 127:94–114.

Chaudron, L. "When and How to Use Mood Stabilizers During Breastfeeding." *Primary Care Update for OB/GYNs* 2000; 7(3).

Chaudron, L., and W. Jefferson. "Mood Stabilizers During Breastfeeding: A Review." *Journal of Clinical Psychiatry* 2000; 61:79–90.

Chaudron, L. H., and Neha Nirodi. "The Obsessive-Compulsive Spectrum in the Perinatal Period: A Prospective Pilot Study." *Archives of Women's Mental Health* March 2010; 1434–1816.

Chiu, C. C., et al. "Omega-3 Fatty Acids for Depression in Pregnancy." *American Journal of Psychiatry* 2003; 160(2):358.

Clark C. T., et al. "Lamotrigine Dosing for Pregnant Patients with Bipolar Disorder." *American Journal of Psychiatry* 2013; 170:1240–7.

Cohen, L. S., et al. "Relapse of Major Depression During Pregnancy in Women Who Maintain or Discontinue Antidepressant Treatment." *The Journal of the American Medical Association* 2006; 295:499–507.

Cohen, L. S., et al. "Venlafaxine in the Treatment of Postpartum Depression." *Journal of Clinical Psychiatry* 2001; 62(8):592–596.

Corral, M., et al. "Morning Light Therapy for Postpartum Depression." *Archives of Women's Mental Health* 2007; 10(5):221–224. Epub 2007 Aug 16.

Cox, J. L., et al. "Detection of Postnatal Depression: Development of the 10-Item Edinburgh Postnatal Depression Scale." *British Journal of Psychiatry* 1987; 150:782–786.

Croen, Lisa A. PhD, et al. "Antidepressant Use During Pregnancy and Childhood Autism Spectrum Disorder." *Archives of General Psychiatry* 2011; 68(11):1104–1112.

Deligiannidis, K. M. and Freeman M. P. "Best Practice in Research." *Clinical Obstetrics and Gynaecology.* 2014 January; 28(1): 85–95.

Derosa, N., and M. C. Logsdon. "A Comparison of Screening Instruments for Depression in Postpartum Adolescents." *Journal of Child and Adolescent Psychiatric Nursing* 2006; 19(1):13–20.

Einarson, A. "Antipsychotic Medication (Safety/Risk) During Pregnancy and Breastfeeding." *Current Women's Health Reviews* 2010, Vol. 6, No. 1.

Einarson, A. "Paroxetine Use in Pregnancy and Increased Risk of Heart Defects." *Canadian Family Physician* 2010 Aug; 56:767–768.

Einarson, A., et al. "Incidence of Major Malformations in Infants Following Antidepressant Exposure in Pregnancy: Results of a Large Prospective Cohort Study." *Canadian Journal of Psychiatry* 2009; 54(4):242–246.

Ersek, J. L., and Larissa Huber. "Physical Activity Prior to and During Pregnancy and Risk of Postpartum Depressive Symptoms." *Journal of Gynecologic & Neonatal Nursing* 2009; 38:556–566.

Field, T. "Postpartum Depression Effects on Early Interactions, Parenting, and Safety Practices: A Review." *Infant Behavior and Development* 2010; 33:1–06.

Field, T., et al. "Prenatal Dysthymia Versus Major Depression Effects on the Neonate." *Infant Behavior and Development* 2008 31:190–193.

Field, T., et al. "Chronic Prenatal Depression and Neonatal Outcome." *International Journal of Neuroscience* 2008; 118:95–103.

Field, Tiffany. "Emotional Care of the At-Risk Infant: Early Interventions for Infants of Depressed Mothers." *Pediatrics* 1998 Nov; 102(5) (suppl):1305–1310.

Field, Tiffany. "Maternal Depression Effects on Infants and Early Interventions." *Preventive Medicine* 1998; 27:200–203.

Fodgkinson, S. C., et al. "Depressive Symptoms and Birth Outcomes among Pregnant Teenagers." *Journal of Pediatric and Adolescent Gynecology* 2010; 23:16–22.

Forman, D. R., et al. "Effective Treatment for Postpartum Depression Is Not Sufficient to Improve the Developing Mother-Child Relationship." *Development and Psychopathology* 2007; 19:585–602.

Freeman, M. P. "Breastfeeding and Antidepressants: Clinical Dilemmas and Expert Perspectives." *Journal of Clinical Psychiatry* 2009; 70:2.

Freeman, M. P. "Omega-3 Fatty Acids: An Ideal Treatment for Depression in Pregnancy?" *Evidence-Based Integrative Medicine* 2003; 1(91):43–49.

Freeman, M.P., et al. "Omega-3 Fatty Acids and Supportive Psychotherapy for Perinatal Depression: A Randomized Placebo-Controlled Study." *Journal of Affective Disorders* 2008; 110(1–2):142–148.

Freeman, M. P., et al. "Postpartum Depression Assessments at Well-Baby Visits: Screening Feasibility, Prevalence, and Risk Factors." *Journal of Women's Health* 2005 Dec; 14(10):929–35.

Gavin, N., et al. "Perinatal Depression Prevalence and Incidence." *Obstetrics & Gynecology* 2005; 106(5).

Gelfland, D., and D. Teti. "The Effects of Maternal Depression on Children." *Clinical Psychology Review* 1990; 10:329–353.

Gjerdingen, D. K., and Barbara P. Yawn. "Postpartum Depression Screening: Importance, Methods, Barriers, and Recommendations for Practice." *Journal of American Board of Family Medicine* 2007; 20:280–288.

Gjerdingen, D. K., et al. "Postpartum Depression Screening at Well-Child Visits: Validity of a 2-Question Screen and the PHQ-9." *Annals of Family Medicine* 2009 Jan-Feb; 7(1):63–70.

Glover, V., and T. G. O'Connor. "Effects of Antenatal Stress and Anxiety: Implications for Development and Psychiatry." *British Journal of Psychiatry* 2002 May; 180:389–391.

Grigoriadis, S., et al. "Antidepressant Exposure During Pregnancy and Congenital Malformations." *Journal of Clinical Psychiatry* 2013; 74:e293–e308.

Grigoriadis, S., et al. "The Effect of Prenatal Antidepressant Exposure on Neonatal Adaptation: A Systematic Review and Meta-Analysis." *Journal of Clinical Psychiatry* 2013; 74:e309.

Grigoriadis, S., et al. "The Impact of Maternal Depression During Pregnancy on Perinatal Outcomes: A Systematic Review and Meta-Analysis." *Journal of Clinical Psychiatry* 2013; 74:e321–e341.

Grzeskowiak, L. E., et al. "Continuation versus Cessation of Antidepressant Use in the Pre- and Post-Natal Period and Impact on Duration of Breastfeeding. Birth Defects Research Part A." *Clinical and Molecular Teratology* 2014; 100:538–539.

Gunlicks, M. L., and M. M. Weissman. "Change in Child Psychopathology With Improvement In Parental Depression: A Systematic Review." *Journal of American Academy of Child and Adolescent Psychiatry* 2008; 47(4):379–389.

Halushka, P. "St. John's Wort: A Mini-Review of its Pharmocokinetics and Anti-Depressant Effects" 12/16/2009. medscape.com/viewarticle/713605.

Hammen, C., and P. A. Brennan. "Severity, Chronicity, and Timing of Maternal Depression and Risk for Adolescent Offspring Diagnoses in a Community Sample." *Archives of General Psychiatry* 2003; 60:253–258.

Hantsoo, Lisa, et al. "A Randomized, Placebo-Controlled, Double-Blind Trial of Sertraline for Postpartum Depression." *Psychopharmacology* 2014; 231:939–948.

Hay, Dale F., et al. "Mothers' Antenatal Depression and Their Children's Antisocial Outcomes." *Child Development* 2010 Jan; 81, No. 1:149–165.

Hendrick, V., and L. Altshuler. "Management of Major Depression During Pregnancy." *American Journal of Psychiatry* 2002 Oct; 159(10):166–173.

Hendrick, V., et al. "Postpartum and Nonpostpartum Depression: Differences in Presentation and Response to Pharmacologic Treatment." *Depression and Anxiety* 2000; 11:66–72.

Hibbeln, J. R. "Seafood Consumption, the DHA Content of Mothers Milk and Prevalence Rates of Postpartum Depression: A Cross-National, Ecological Analysis." *Journal of Affective Disorders* 2001.

Hviid, A., et al. "Use of Selective Serotonin Reuptake Inhibitors During Pregnancy and Risk of Autism." *New England Journal of Medicine* 2013; 369:2406–15.

Jain, A. I., and Timothy Lacy. "Psychotropic Drugs in Pregnancy and Lactation." *Journal of Psychiatric Practice* 2005; 11:177–191.

Jaques, S. C., et al. "Cannabis, the Pregnant Woman and Her Child." *Journal of Perinatology* 2014; 34(6):417424.

Kelly, Lauren E., et al. "Neonatal Benzodiazepines Exposure during Breastfeeding." *The Journal of Pediatrics* September 2012; 161, (3): 448–451.

Kendall-Tackett, K., et al. "Depression, Sleep Quality, and Maternal Well-Being in Postpartum Women with a History of Sexual Assault: A Comparison of Breastfeeding, Mixed-Feeding, and Formula-Feeding Mothers." *Breastfeeding Medicine* 2013; 8(1):16-22.

Koren G., and H. Nordeng. "Antidepressant Use During Pregnancy: The Benefit-Risk Ratio." *American Journal of Obstetrics and Gynecology* 2012; 207:157–163.

Koren, G., et al. "Is Maternal Use of Selective Serotonin Reuptake Inhibitors in the Third Trimester of Pregnancy Harmful to Neonates?" *Canadian Medical Association Journal* 2005; 172(11).

Lerandowski, R. E., et al. "Predictors of Positive Outcomes in Offspring of Depressed Parents and Non-depressed Parents Across 20 Years." *Journal of Child and Family Studies* 2014; 23:800–811.

Lindahl, V., et al. "Prevalence of Suicidality During Pregnancy and the Postpartum." *Archives of Women's Mental Health* 2005; 8:77–87.

Louik, C., et al. "First-Trimester Use of Selective Serotonin-Reuptake Inhibitors and the Risk of Birth Defects." *New England Journal of Medicine* 2007; 356:2675–2683.

Malm. H., et al. "Risks Associated With Selective Serotonin Reuptake Inhibitors in Pregnancy." *American Journal of Obstetrics and Gynecology* 2005; 106:1289–1296.

Manber, R., et al. "Acupuncture for Depression During Pregnancy." *American Journal of Obstetrics and Gynecology* 2010; 115:511–520.

Marcus, S. M. "Depression During Pregnancy: Rates, Risks and Consequences." *The Canadian Journal of Clinical Pharmacology* Winter 2009;16 (1):e15–e22.

Marcus, S. M., et al. "Depressive Symptoms Among Pregnant Women Screened in Obstetric Settings." *Journal of Women's Health* 2003; 12(4):373–380.

Maschi, S., et al. "Neonatal Outcome Following Pregnancy Exposure to Antidepressants: A Prospective Controlled Cohort Study." *British Journal of Obstetrics and Gynaecology* 2008; 115:283–289.

McKenna, K., et al. "Pregnancy Outcome of Women Using Atypical Antipsychotic Drugs: A Prospective Comparative Study." *Journal of Clinical Psychiatry* 2005; 66:444–449.

Meador, K. J., et al. "Cognitive Function at 3 Years of Age after Fetal Exposure to Antiepileptic Drugs." *New England Journal of Medicine* 2009; 360(16):1597–1605.

Misri, S. "Managing Unipolar Depression in Pregnancy." *Current Opinion in Psychiatry* 2009; 22(1):13–18.

Moretti, M. E., et al. "Evaluating the Safety of St. John's Wort in Human Pregnancy." *Reproductive Toxicology* 2009; 28(1):96–99.

Moses-Kolko, E. L., et al. "Neonatal Signs After Late In Utero Exposure to Serotonin Reuptake Inhibitors: Literature Review and Implications for Clinical Applications." *Journal of American Medical Association* 2005; 293(19):2372–2383.

Moses-Kolko, E. L., et al. "Transdermal Estradiol for Postpartum Depression: A Promising Treatment Option." *Clinical Obstetrics and Gynecology* 2009; 52(3):516–529.

Mounts, K. O. "Screening for Maternal Depression in the Neonatal ICU." *Clinical Perinatology* 2009; 36:137–152.

Mulcahy, R., et al. "A Randomised Control Trial for the Effectiveness of Group Interpersonal Psychotherapy for Postnatal Depression." *Archives of Women's Mental Health* 2010; 13:125–139.

Muzik, M., and Stefana Borovska. "Perinatal Depression: Implications for Child Mental Health." *Mental Health in Family Medicine* 2010; 7:239-47.

Newport, D. J., et al. "Lamotrigine in Breast Milk and Nursing Infants: Determination of Exposure." *Pediatrics* 2008; 122(1). http://www.pediatrics.Org/cgi/content/full/122/l/e223.

Newport, D. J., et al. "The Treatment of Postpartum Depression: Minimizing Infant Exposures." *Journal of Clinical Psychiatry* 2002; 63 (suppl 7):31–44.

Nonacs, R., and L. S. Cohen. "Depression During Pregnancy: Diagnosis and Treatment Options." *Journal of Clinical Psychiatry* 2002; 63 (suppl 7):24–30.

Nonacs, R., and L. S. Cohen. "Postpartum Mood Disorders: Diagnosis and Treatment Guidelines." *Journal of Clinical Psychiatry* 1998; 59 (suppl 2):34–40.

Nordeng, F. L., and O. Spigset. "Treatment with Selective Serotonin Reuptake Inhibitors in the Third Trimester of Pregnancy: Effects on the Infant." *Drug Safe* 2005; 28(7):565–581.

Norman, E., et al. "An Exercise and Education Program Improves Wellbeing of New Mothers: A Randomized Controlled Trial." *Physical Therapy* 2010; 90:348–355.

Nulman, I., et al. "Child Development Following Exposure to Tricyclic Antidepressants or Fluoxetine Throughout Fetal Life: A Prospective, Controlled Study." *American Journal of Psychiatry* 2002 Nov; 159:1889–1895.

Nulman, I., et al. "Neurodevelopment of Children Exposed In Utero to Antidepressant Drugs." *New England Journal of Medicine* 1997; 336(4):258–262.

Nulman I., et al. "Neurodevelopment of Children Following Prenatal Exposure to Venlafaxine, Selective Serotonin Reuptake Inhibitors, or Untreated Maternal Depression." *American Journal of Psychiatry* 2012; 169:1165.

Oates, M. "Perinatal Psychiatric Disorders: A Leading Cause of Maternal Morbidity and Mortality." *British Medical Bulletin* 2003; 67:219–229.

Occhiogrosso, M., et al. "Persistent Pulmonary Hypertension of the Newborn and Selective Serotonin Reuptake Inhibitors: Lessons from Clinical and Translational Studies." *American Journal of Psychiatry* 2012; 169:134–140.

O'Hara, M. W., et al. "Efficacy of Interpersonal Psychotherapy for Postpartum Depression." *Archives of General Psychiatry* 2000; 57(11):1039–1045.

Oren, D. A., et al. "An Open Trial of Morning Light Therapy for Treatment of Antepartum Depression." *American Journal of Psychiatry* 2002 Apr; 159(4):666–669.

Orr, S. T., et al. "Maternal Prenatal Depressive Symptoms and Spontaneous Preterm Births Among African-American Women in

Baltimore, Maryland." *American Journal of Epidemiology*. 2002; 156:797–802.

Palladino, C., et al. "Homicide and Suicide During the Perinatal Period." *American Journal of Obstetrics and Gynecology* 2011; 118:1056–63.

Paulson, J. F., and Sharnail D. Bazemore. "Prenatal and Postpartum Depression in Fathers and Association with Maternal Depression: A Meta-Analysis." *Journal of American Medical Association* 2010; 303(19):1961–1969.

Paulson, J. F., et al. "Individual and Combined Effects of Postpartum Depression in Mothers and Fathers on Parenting Behavior." *Pediatrics* Aug 2006:118(2); 659–668.

Pedersen, L. H., et al. "Prenatal Antidepressant Exposure and Behavioral Problems in Early Childhood—A Cohort Study." *Acta Psychiatrica Scandinavica* 2013; 127–126.

Pinelli, J. M., et al. "Case Report and Review of the Perinatal Implications of Maternal Lithium Use." *American Journal of Obstetrics and Gynecology* 2002 Jul; 187(1):245–249.

Pinheiro, Emily, et al. "Sertraline and Breastfeeding: Review and Meta-Analysis." *Achives of Women's Mental Health*. April 2015, Volume 18, Issue 2, pp 139–146.

Pope, C. J., et al. "Recognition, Diagnosis and Treatment of Postpartum Bipolar Depression." *Expert Review of Neurotherapeutics* 2014. 14(1), 19–28 (2014)

Ramchandani, P. G., et al. "Depression in Men in the Postnatal Period and Later Child Psychopathology: A Population Cohort Study." *Journal of American Academy of Child and Adolecscent Psychiatry* 2008; 47:390–398.

Reck C. K., et al. "Prevalence, Onset and Comorbidity of Postpartum Anxiety and Depressive Disorders." *Acta Psychiatrica Scandinavica* 2008; 118:459–468.

Robinson, G. E. "Controversies About the Use of Antidepressants in Pregnancy." *Journal of Nervous and Mental Disease* March 2015.:203(3):159–163.

Ross L. E, et al. "Selected Pregnancy and Delivery Outcomes After Exposure to Antidepressant Medication: A Systematic Review and Meta-Analysis." *Journal of American Medical Association Psychiatry* 2013; 70:436–443.

Ross, L., et al. "Sleep and Perinatal Mood Disorders: A Critical Review." *Journal of Psychiatry and Neuroscience* 2005; 30(4).

Russell, E., et al. "Risk of Obsessive-Compulsive Disorder in Pregnant and Postpartum Women: A Meta-Analysis." *Journal of Clinical Psychiatry* 2013; 74(4), 377–385

Sanz, E. J., et al. "Selective Serotonin Reuptake Inhibitors in Pregnant Women and Neonatal Withdrawal Syndrome Database Analysis" (see comment). *Lancet* 2005; 356(9458):482–487.

Segre, L. S., et al. "Interpersonal Psychotherapy for Antenatal and Postpartum Depression." *Primary Psychiatry* 2004; 11(3):52–56.

Sharma, V., et al. "Bipolar II Postpartum Depression: Detection, Diagnosis, and Treatment." *American Journal of Psychiatry* 2009; 166:1217–1221.

Shaw, R. J., et al. "The Relationship Between Acute Stress Disorder and Posttraumatic Stress Disorder in the Neonatal Intensive Care Unit." *Psychosomatics* 2009; 50:131–137.

Sidebottom, A. C., et al. "Validation of the Patient Health Questionnaire (PHQ)-9 for Prenatal Depression Screening." *Archives of Women's Mental Health* 2012; 15:367–374.

Sit, D., and Katherine L. Wisner. "Identification of Postpartum Depression." *Clinical Obstetrics and Gynecology* 2009 Sep; 52(3):456–468.

Smit, M., et al. "Mirtazapine in Pregnancy and Lactation: Data from a Case Series." *Journal of Clinical Psychopharmacology* 2015 Feb 13.

Sorensen, M. J., et al. "Antidepressant Exposure in Pregnancy and Risk of Autism Spectrum Disorder." *Clinical Epidemiology* 2013; 5:449-559.

Spinelli, M. G. "Interpersonal Psychotherapy for Depressed Antepartum Women: A Pilot Study." *American Journal of Psychiatry* 1997; 154:1028–1030.

Spinelli, M. G., and J. Endicott. "Controlled Clinical Trial of Interpersonal Psychotherapy Versus Parenting Education Program for Depressed Pregnant Women." *American Journal of Psychiatry* 2003; 160(3):555–562.

Stowe, Z. N., and C. B. Nemeroff. "Women at Risk for Postpartum-Onset Major Depression." *American Journal of Obstetrics and Gynecology* 1995 Aug; 173(2):639–644.

Stowe, Z., et al. "Paroxetine in Human Breast Milk and Nursing Infants." *American Journal of Psychiatry* 2000; 157:185–189.

Stuart, S., et al. "The Prevention and Psychotherapeutic Treatment of Postpartum Depression." *Archives of Women's Mental Health* 2003; 6 (suppl 2):57–59.

Suri, R., et al. "Effects of Antenatal Depression and Antidepressant Treatment on Gestational Age at Birth and Risk of Preterm Birth." *American Journal of Psychiatry* 2007; 164:1206–1213.

Suri, R. A., et al. "Managing Psychiatric Medications in the Breastfeeding Woman." *Medscape Women's Health* 1998; 3(1).

Tam, L. W., et al. "Screening Women for Postpartum Depression at Well Baby Visits: Resistance Encountered and Recommendations." *Archives of Women's Mental Health* 2002; 5:79–82.

Van den Bergh, B. R., et al. "Antenatal Maternal Anxiety and Stress and the Neurobehavioral Development of the Fetus and Child: Links and Possible Mechanisms. A Review." *Neuroscience & Biobehavioral Reviews* 2005 Apr; 29(2):237–58.

Viguera, A. C., et al. "Risk of Recurrence in Women with Bipolar Disorder During Pregnancy: Prospective Study of Mood Stabilizer Discontinuation." *American Journal of Psychiatry* 2007; 164:1817–1824.

Warburton, W., et al. "A Register Study of the Impact of Stopping Third Trimester Selective Serotonin Reuptake Inhibitor Exposure on Neonatal Health." *Acta Psychiatrica Scandinavica* 2009; 1–9.

Weissmann, A. M., et al. "Pooled Analysis of Antidepressant Levels in Lactating Mothers, Breast Milk, and Nursing Infants." *American Journal of Psychiatry* 2004; 161:1066–1078.

Wilson, K. L., et al. "Persistent Pulmonary Hypertension of the Newborn Is Associated with Mode of Delivery and Not with Maternal Use of Selective Serotonin Reuptake Inhibitors." *American Journal of Perinatology* 2010: Jul.

Wisner, K. L. "Prevention of Recurrent Postpartum Depression: A Randomized Clinical Trial." *Journal of Clinical Psychiatry* 2001 Feb; 62(2):82–86.

Wisner, K. L. "Timing of Depression Recurrence in the First Year After Birth." *Journal of Affective Disorders* 2004; 78(3):249–52.

Wisner, K. L., and C. Schaefer. "Psychotropic Drugs," in *Drugs During Pregnancy and Lactation: Treatment Options and Risk Assessment. Academic Press* 2015; 293–339.

Wisner, K. L., et al. "Antidepressant Treatment During Breastfeeding." *American Journal of Psychiatry* 1996; 153(9):1132–1137.

Wisner, K. L., et al. "Major Depression and Antidepressant Treatment: Impact on Pregnancy and Neonatal Outcomes Medications and Lactation." *American Journal of Psychiatry in Advance* 2009; 166:557–566.

Wisner, K. L., et al. "Onset Timing, Thoughts of Self-harm, and Diagnoses in Postpartum Women with Screen-Positive Depression Findings." *Journal of American Medicine Psychiatry*, published online March 2013.

Yonkers, K., et al. "Management of Bipolar Disorder During Pregnancy The Postpartum Period." *Focus* 2005; 3:266–279.

Yonkers, K. A., et al. "The Management of Depression During Pregnancy: A Report from the American Psychiatric Association and the American College of Obstetricians and Gynecologists." *General Hospital Psychiatry* 2009; 31:403–413.

Appendix

Medical Terms

bipolar disorder—Also known as manic depression, bipolar disorder is characterized by mood swings from manic (see "mania") to depressed. Many researchers believe there is a strong genetic component to this illness. Bipolar disorder occurs on a spectrum of severity. Bipolar I includes repeated episodes of mania and depression. Bipolar II is characterized by recurrent periods of hypomania and depression. Manic episodes can include hallucinations and delusions, which create a medical emergency. Hypomanic swings can include trouble sleeping, irritability, agitation/anxiety, and difficulty concentrating. Often people are considered "moody." Often there is a history of a family member (who may never have been diagnosed) with bipolar disorder.

cognitive behavioral therapy (CBT)—Cognitive behavioral therapy has been well researched and shown to be a very effective form of psychotherapy for perinatal issues.

With CBT, the therapist takes an active role in the therapy process and provides a clear structure and focus to treatment. Cognitive therapy teaches the client how certain thought patterns, beliefs, and behaviors create symptoms such as depression, anxiety, or anger. The therapist works with the client to help develop new positive ways of thinking and acting. CBT encourages and supports the client in creating specific, practical goals, and techniques to achieve them. The focus is on creating new skills.

cortisol—Called the "stress hormone," cortisol is a hormone released by the adrenal glands during anxious or agitated states.

delusion—This is a false belief. A person may fear being chased or spied on or think she is someone other than herself. Often there is religious content to the thoughts.

depression—A common disorder characterized by sad mood, irritability, sleep and appetite disturbances, loss of pleasure, fatigue, and hopelessness. Depression can be caused by a variety of factors, including biochemical, emotional, and psychological.

etiology—The cause or origin of a disease or illness.

hallucination—Something a person sees (visual hallucination) or hears (auditory hallucination) that others do not. Hallucinations often have religious overtones, for example, hearing the voice of God or Satan. These hallucinations often include commands, telling the woman she should do certain things.

hypomania—Sometimes confused with the normal joy and excitation of having a new baby, hypomanic symptoms include increased goal-directed activity, being overly talkative, racing thoughts, decreased need for sleep, distractibility, and irritability. There is no significant difficulty with functioning, but hypomania is associated with significant depression later in the postpartum period.

insomnia—Inability to sleep. This can be trouble falling or staying asleep.

interpersonal psychotherapy (IPT)—IPT is a brief and highly structured psychotherapy that addresses interpersonal issues. This model of therapy has been shown to be effective for prenatal and postpartum mood and anxiety disorders.

IPT helps the client solve problems, for instance, disagreements, feeling isolated, adjusting to new roles, or grief following a loss. The therapist works from a collaborative framework.

mania—A symptom of bipolar disorder (see above) characterized by exaggerated excitement, hyperactivity, and racing, scattered thoughts. A person in a manic state feels an emotional "high" and often does not use good judgment. Speech may be rapid and she may feel little need for sleep or food. Thinking is usually confused, and she may act in sexually, socially, and physically unhealthy ways, for instance, inappropriate sexual behavior or shopping sprees.

mood instability—When moods change rapidly. Mood may swing from happy to sad, for instance.

neurotransmitter—Chemical released by nerve cells that carries information from one cell to another. This type of chemical transmits messages in the brain. Some neurotransmitters are serotonin, norepinephrine, and dopamine.

obsessive-compulsive disorder (OCD)—Occurs in about 1 in 100 people. OCD is associated with a chemical imbalance in the brain. This condition worsens in times of stress. Obsessions are thoughts that occur intrusively (they seem to just appear) and repetitively (over and over again). Even with reassurance, people with obsessions continue to worry or have repetitive thoughts. Compulsions are repetitive actions taken to reduce anxiety produced by the obsession. Compulsions often take the form of cleaning, checking (for instance, the locks on the door or the baby's breathing), or counting (for instance, the number of diapers in the bag). A person may have only obsessions, or obsessions and compulsions.

panic disorder—During a panic attack, the person may feel symptoms including intense fear, rapid breathing, sweating, nausea, dizziness, and numbness or tingling. Sufferers often fear having the next panic attack and may develop behaviors to avoid situations they think put them at risk.

perinatal mood or anxiety disorder —A mood disorder (for instance, depression) or anxiety disorder (for example, panic) beginning during pregnancy or during the first year postpartum.

phobia—A persistent, irrational fear of a specific object, activity, or situation. This fear usually leads either to avoidance of the feared object or situation, or to experiencing it with dread. Common phobias include fear of heights, flying in airplanes, small places, and spiders.

postpartum—After a mother gives birth. An illness is considered postpartum if it begins in the first year after birth.

post-traumatic stress disorder (PTSD) —PTSD can occur following life-threatening or injury- producing events such as sexual abuse or assault, or traumatic childbirth. People who suffer from PTSD often experience nightmares and flashbacks, have difficulty sleeping, and feel detached. Symptoms can be severe and significantly impair daily life. Observers of trauma can also develop PTSD.

premenstrual dysphoric disorder (PMDD) —A combination of symptoms that appear a week or two before a menstrual period, and go away within a week after the onset of the period. Common symptoms include bloating, cramping, irritability, fatigue, anger, and depression. About 75 percent of women experience some degree of premenstrual mood symptoms.

prenatal—During pregnancy.

psychoanalysis—A form of psychotherapy that focuses on unconscious factors affecting current relationships and patterns of behavior, traces the factors to their origins, shows how they have changed over time, and helps the client cope with adult life. The client talks and the therapist is primarily a listener. Usually therapy takes place four or five times a week, and can continue for years. This is the kind of therapy that's often shown in movies or on television.

psychosis—An extreme and potentially dangerous mental disturbance that includes losing touch with reality. The psychotic person displays irrational behavior and has hallucinations and delusions. Hospitalization and medication are required. It is now thought most postpartum psychosis is due to bipolar illness. Women with psychosis have a higher rate of suicide and infanticide (killing the infant) as a result.

psychotropic medication—Medication that affects thought processes or feeling states by acting on brain chemistry. Antidepressants and antianxiety medications are included in this category.

relapse—To become ill again, after a period of wellness.

Healthcare Professionals

Note: Licensure varies from state to state. Also, information about perinatal mood disorders is not a routine part of most training programs. See the section in Chapter 3 on finding a knowledgeable therapist or psychiatrist.

certified midwife (CM)—A CM is an individual educated in the discipline of midwifery, who is certified by the American College of Nurse-Midwives. The CM provides primary healthcare to women, including prenatal care, labor and delivery care, care after birth, gynecological exams, newborn care, assistance with family planning, pre-conception care, menopausal management, and counseling in health maintenance.

certified nurse- midwife (CNM)—A CNM is a licensed healthcare practitioner educated in nursing and midwifery. She provides primary healthcare to women of childbearing age, including prenatal care, labor and delivery care, care after birth, gynecological exams, newborn care, assistance with family planning, pre-pregnancy care, menopausal management, and counseling in health maintenance. CNMs attend over 9 percent of the births in the United States. Many CNMs are able to prescribe medication.

clinical psychologist—Mental health professionals who have earned a doctoral degree in psychology (either a PhD, PsyD, or EdD). They have received extensive clinical training in research, assessment, and the application of different psychological therapies. Clinical psychologists are concerned with the study, diagnosis, treatment, and prevention of mental and emotional disorders. They are not able to prescribe medication.

doula, birth doula—The word *doula* is derived from a Greek word that translates "woman's servant." The certified birth doulas role is to provide physical and emotional support to women and their partners during labor and birth. Birth doulas do not perform clinical tasks such as vaginal exams or fetal heart rate monitoring. Doulas are not trained to diagnose medical or psychological conditions or give medical advice; rather they help women advocate for their birth preferences. Birth doulas educate women regarding physical and emotional comfort measures for labor, birth, and the immediate postpartum period, including initial breastfeeding.

doula, postpartum—There is a difference between a birth doula and a postpartum doula. Postpartum doulas provide physical, emotional, and educational support for women and partners after the baby comes home. Certified postpartum doulas are infant CPR certified, and trained in lactation support, newborn care, nutrition, and emotional adjustment to parenthood in the first weeks of the baby's life. Postpartum doulas will often offer light housework and meal preparation. For more information about certifying agencies, see the Resources section.

Questions to help you select a doula:

Are you certified?

Are you trained in postpartum depression?

What is your view regarding use of medication for depression?

What are the local resources you can help us with regarding postpartum depression?

endocrinologist—A physician (MD) who specializes in treating problems related to hormones. Endocrinologists frequently treat thyroid problems.

lactation consultant—Trained, often certified, specialist who provides support and education about the process of breastfeeding. A lactation consultant can provide help regarding nursing, pumping, bottlefeeding, and weaning.

licensed clinical professional counselor (LCPC)—An LCPC is a masters-level mental health professional. LCPCs are not able to prescribe medications.

marriage and family therapist (MFT)—A professional with a master's-level license, MFTs are similar to LCSWs and LCPCs. They are trained in individual, couple, and family therapy. MFTs are not able to prescribe medication.

midwives, other—(See "certified nurse-midwife" and "certified midwife.") Some women practice midwifery without a license. Be sure to ask about training and licensure.

psychiatric nurse (APRN)—Registered nurses who seek additional education and obtain a masters or doctoral degree can become advanced practice registered nurses in a specialty (APRNs). They provide the full range of psychiatric care services to individuals, families, groups, and communities, and in most states they have the authority to prescribe medications. APRNs are qualified to practice independently.

psychiatric social worker—These mental health professionals have earned the MSW (masters in social work) degree and are trained to be sensitive to the impact of environmental factors on mental disorders. LCSW designates licensed clinical social worker. These professionals cannot prescribe medication.

psychiatrist—These mental health professionals have earned the MD (medical doctor) degree. Advanced training focuses on psychiatric diagnosis, psychopharmacology (medication management of mental health issues), and psychotherapy. These physicians are the experts in prescribing psychotropic medications.

psychotherapist—A person who practices psychotherapy: either a clinical psychologist, psychiatrist, professional counselor, social worker, or other mental health professional. Only a medical doctor, clinical nurse specialist, or physician assistant can prescribe medication.

Endorsements and Awards

Beyond the Blues is a recommended resource by many professionals, organizations, agencies and educational institutions including:

Brooke Shields, actress and author on Postpartum Depression
Childbirth and Postpartum Professional Association (CAPPA)
Durham Regional Health Department of Canada
First 5 Butte County, California
International Childbirth Education Association. (ICEA)
Michigan Spectrum Health
New York State Department of Health
Pine Rest Christian Mental Health Services
Postpartum Support International (PSI)
Rex Health Center, University of North Carolina
United States Department of Health and Human Services
U.S. Navy

Awards include:

iParenting Media Award
Gold Award, National Parenting Publications
Bronze Award, National Health Information

Seminars, Training, Workshops, and Consultation

Drs. Bennett and Indman offer consultation, lectures, and training on perinatal illness to a wide variety of professionals and organizations. Sample topics include:

- Assessment, diagnosis, and prevention
- Psychotherapy models and techniques
- The latest research in psychopharmacology
- Consequences of untreated illness
- Resources to help suffering families.

They tailor their presentations to fit the particular needs and interests of the participants. Working individually or as a team, they can provide any type of program at your facility, from a brief lunch hour talk to a comprehensive two-day seminar. Please contact them directly for scheduling and fee information.

Contact Shoshana Bennett or Pec Indman directly:

SHOSHANA BENNETT, PHD

DrShosh@DrShosh.com

510-305-5040

PEC INDMAN EDD, MFT

pec@beyondtheblues.com

408-255-1730

About the Authors

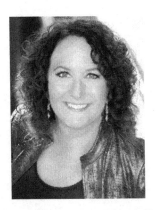

SHOSHANA BENNETT, PHD ("Dr. Shosh"), the mother of Elana and Aaron, founded Postpartum Assistance for Mothers in 1987 after her second experience with two life-threatening postpartum depressions. She is the author of *Children of the Depressed, Pregnant on Prozac* and *Postpartum Depression for Dummies*. National TV shows feature Dr. Shosh as the postpartum expert, and news stations consult her. She's interviewed regularly on national radio and has been quoted in dozens of newspapers and magazines. She is a past president of Postpartum Support International, noted guest lecturer, and keynote speaker. Dr. Shosh developed PPDGone!, the first app for perinatal illness, and she's an Executive Producer of the film *Dark Side of the Full Moon*. She earned three teaching credentials, two master's degrees, a PhD, and is licensed as a clinical psychologist.

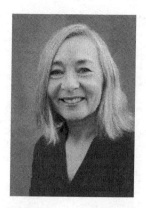

PEC INDMAN, EDD, MFT, has a doctorate in counseling and a master's degree in health psychology, and is licensed as a marriage and family therapist. Her training as a physician assistant in family practice was at Johns Hopkins University. Dr. Indman is the Past Chair of Education and Training for Postpartum Support International. She is active in the North American Society for Psychosocial OB/GYN and the Marcé Society, and participates in annual conferences. Dr. Indman has been interviewed on national radio and international and national television and for magazines and newspapers. Lecturing for a wide variety of audiences nationally and internationally, Dr. Indman has served as an expert advisor for federal and local programs. She is in private practice in San Jose, California, and is the mother of two girls, Megan and Emily.

Index

Made in the USA
Middletown, DE
04 June 2016